Stains and
Staining Procedures in
MICROBIOLOGY

Stains and
Staining Procedures in
MICROBIOLOGY

BS Nagoba MSc, PhD (Medical Microbiology)
Professor, Department of Microbiology and
Assistant Dean (R&D),
MIMSR Medical College, Latur

Megha Rastogi MD (Microbiology)
Department of Microbiology
MIMSR Medical College, Latur

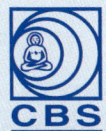

CBS Publishers & Distributors Pvt Ltd

New Delhi • Bengaluru • Chennai • Kochi • Kolkata • Mumbai
Hyderabad • Nagpur • Patna • Pune • Vijayawada

Stains and Staining
Procedures in
MICROBIOLOGY

ISBN: 978-93-86310-82-8

First Edition: 2017

Published by Satish Kumar Jain and produced by Varun Jain for

CBS Publishers & Distributors Pvt Ltd

4819/XI Prahlad Street, 24 Ansari Road, Daryaganj, New Delhi 110 002, India.
Ph: 23289259, 23266861, 23266867 Website: www.cbspd.com
Fax: 011-23243014   e-mail: delhi@cbspd.com; cbspubs@airtelmail.in.

Corporate Office: 204 FIE, Industrial Area, Patparganj, Delhi 110 092

Ph: 4934 4934   Fax: 4934 4935   e-mail: publishing@cbspd.com; publicity@cbspd.com

Branches

- **Bengaluru:** Seema House 2975, 17th Cross, K.R. Road,
  Banasankari 2nd Stage, Bengaluru 560 070, Karnataka
  Ph: +91-80-26771678/79   Fax: +91-80-26771680   e-mail: bangalore@cbspd.com
- **Chennai:** 7, Subbaraya Street, Shenoy Nagar, Chennai 600 030, Tamil Nadu
  Ph: +91-44-26680620, 26681266   Fax: +91-44-42032115   e-mail: chennai@cbspd.com
- **Kochi:** Ashana House, No. 39/1904, AM Thomas Road, Valanjambalam,
  Ernakulam 682 016, Kochi, Kerala
  Ph: +91-484-4059061-65   Fax: +91-484-4059065   e-mail: kochi@cbspd.com
- **Kolkata:** 6/B, Ground Floor, Rameswar Shaw Road, Kolkata-700 014, West Bengal
  Ph: +91-33-22891126, 22891127, 22891128   e-mail: kolkata@cbspd.com
- **Mumbai:** 83-C, Dr E Moses Road, Worli, Mumbai-400018, Maharashtra
  Ph: +91-22-24902340/41   Fax: +91-22-24902342   e-mail: mumbai@cbspd.com

Representatives

- **Hyderabad** 0-9885175004 • **Nagpur**   0-9021734563 • **Patna** 0-9334159340
- **Pune**   0-9623451994 • **Vijayawada** 0-9000660880

Printed at Paras Offset Pvt. Ltd., New Delhi, India

Preface

This book has been exclusively written for the postgraduate students in microbiology, pathology and biotechnology to provide different staining procedures in microbiology under one roof.

An attempt has been made to cover the details of almost all staining procedures used for the demonstration of different groups of microorganisms. Sincere efforts have been made to offer a text that is accurate, concise, easy to understand, uptodate and user friendly with relevant diagrams. A special care has been taken to give detailed information wherever necessary.

Though this book has been exclusively designed for the post-graduate students in microbiology, pathology and biotechno-logy, it will be of help to postgraduates students in parasitology, mycology, botany, zoology and other courses such as DMLT, pharmacy, etc. to understand the various stains and staining procedures in microbiology.

We hope this book will receive attention and appreciation from postgraduate students and teachers and will prove very useful for them to practice the different staining procedures routinely. Though efforts have been taken to cover all minute details, we do not claim perfection. We are open for discussion and welcome your constructive suggestions to make this book more perfect in subsequent editions.

BS Nagoba
Megha Rastogi

Acknowledgements

We are very happy to express our gratitude to Hon. Prof. Dr VD Karad, Executive President and Director General, MAEER's MIT, Pune, a dynamic personality and a renowned educationalist. He has always been a source of inspiration, guidance and help to us.

We are thankful to Shri RK Karad, Executive Director and Dr Mrs Sarita Mantri, Principal, MIMSR Medical College, Latur, for their support and guidance.

A very special thanks are due to Dr Nashira Shaikh, Associate Professor, Microbiology, Dr VM Medical College, Solapur, for mycology figures, Miss Pallavi Nagoba, Miss Ramani Nagoba and Mr JB Mule for drawing figures.

We are also thankful to Dr AP Pichare, Dr AR Lamture, Mr PB Kendre, Dr SM Dharne, Dr Milind Dawane, Dr SV Munde and other colleagues in the Dept of Microbiology, MIMSR Medical College, Latur, for their support and cooperation.

We would like to thank Senior Librarian Mr VN Kale, Miss Namita Surwase, Mr Dayanand Ghante, Mr Pandurang Jadhav, Mr Vinod Jogdand, Mr VP Mane, Mr Gaurav Mule, Mr Pangaonkar and Mr Gore for their sustained efforts in the preparation of manuscript.

We are also thankful to Mr SS Gutte, Mr Datta Shinde, Mr MJ Kaule and Mr SS Kadam for their timely help.

Finally we would like to thank CBS Publishers Pvt. Ltd, in particular Mr Javed and Mr Arjuna for their cooperation and sustained efforts in the publication of this book.

BS Nagoba
Megha Rastogi

Contents

Introduction to Stains

WHY ARE STAINS NECESSARY?

- Microbes are semitransparent or transparent; hence, difficult to visualize in unstained state/preparations. This is because of very little contrast obtained between their cells and surrounding medium, as the surrounding medium is transparent/semitransparent.

- Microorganisms become nearly opaque when they are stained. Thus, staining increases the contrast between microbes and surrounding medium as the surrounding medium remains transparent or semitransparent. Ultimately, the result is clear visualization of microbes under the microscope. Thus, stains help:
  - To render microscopic and semitransparent objects visible, e.g. bacteria, fungi, parasites, viruses and other cell types such as pus cells, epithelial cells, etc.
  - To reveal their size and shape.
  - To study the various internal and external structures—intracellular structures like spores and extracellular structures like capsule.
  - To produce specific physical and chemical reactions.
  - To study chemical nature of the cells.

- To study classification and identification of microbes—presence of certain structures and staining reactions aid in identification and classification.

STAIN AND DYE

Stain

It is a substance that adheres to cell and colours the cell. It is a more purified colouring agent that is to be used for biological purpose.

Dye

- It is a less purified colouring agent that itself is coloured and used for general purpose.
- The two terms, dye and stains are used interchangeably by the biologists, but they are not the same. Colouring agent that is to be used for general purpose is called dye and one that is to be used for biological purpose is called a stain.
- Dyes are less purified preparations and are satisfactory for colouring in textile industries (textile colouring agents), while stains are more purified preparations and are manufactured with greater care under more rigid specifications so that they are satisfactory for the procedures in which they are employed.
- Dyes are of two types:
    1. *Natural:* Predominated during early years.
    2. *Artificial and synthetic:* These are commonly used nowadays. Majority of the dyes used in microbiology are of synthetic type.
        – Some of them are derived from aniline dyes and are referred as **aniline dyes** (manufactured from aniline, which is derived from nitrobenzene).
        – Many of them are derived from coal tar and are more correctly referred as **coal tar dyes** as all of them are derived from one or more substances found in coal tar.
        – The coal tar dyes are classified as acidic and basic dyes.

Definition of Dye/Stain and Staining

- According to Conn et al., dye or stain can be defined as an organic compound containing both chromophoric and auxophoric groups linked to a benzene ring.

- A **chromophoric** group imparts to the compound the property of colour and **auxophoric** group imparts to the compound the property of electrolytic dissociation, i.e. salt forming property.
- To be a stain/dye, the presence of both chromophoric and auxophoric groups is essential.
- Compounds of benzene containing chromophore radicals are known as **chromogens**.
- Chromogens, although coloured, are not dyes because they do not possess auxophores and hence, do not have affinity and ability to unite.

Staining

It is a procedure in which coloured chemicals called dyes/stains are added to smears/films. Dyes/stains impart a colour to cells or parts of cells by becoming affixed to them through a chemical reaction.

ACIDIC, BASIC AND NEUTRAL DYES

- Dyes are of two types—acidic and basic.
- The distinction between acidic and basic dyes depends on whether the dye portion of the molecule, has a positive or negative electrical charge.

i. Acidic Dyes

- Dyes which ionize to the dye portion of the molecule, a negative charge (ionize to give negative electric charge).
- These are salts of coloured acids like sodium, potassium, calcium and ammonium salts.
- The colouring component is contained in the acidic radical and the base part of stain is colourless, i.e. they contain a coloured negative ion and a colourless positive ion. They have affinity for components of cell which are alkaline in nature.
- They are not frequently used in microbiology, except for background staining. Cytoplasm is usually stained by acidic stain.

- The structures stained by acidic dyes are called acidophilic and those stained by eosin are called eosinophilic.
- Examples: Eosin, acid fuchsin, and nigrosin.

ii. Basic Dyes

- Dyes which ionize to the dye portion of the molecule a positive charge (ionize to give positive electric charge).
- These are salts of coloured bases of chlorides, sometimes sulfate/acetate.
- The colouring component is contained in the basic radical and the acidic part of stain is colourless, i.e. they contain a coloured positive ion and a colourless negative ion.
- They have affinity for cell structures that are acidic in nature.
- They are most commonly used stains in microbiology. They are used to stain nuclei and metachromatic granules.
- The structures which are stained by basic dyes are called as basophilic.
- Examples: Crystal violet, methylene blue, malachite green, safranine, etc.

iii. Neutral (Compound) Dyes

- Neutral dye, which is also known as compound dye, is a mixture of two dyes, i.e. when a basic dye is mixed with an acidic dye then a compound dye is formed in which a basic dye contains coloured cations while acidic dye contains coloured anions. Thus, in neutral dyes both acidic and basic components are coloured.
- These dyes are usually formed from the precipitate, which is produced when aqueous acidic and basic dyes combine.
- They are soluble in alcohol and insoluble in water. They stain nucleic acid as well as the cytoplasm. Nuclei are stained by basic dye and cytoplasm by acidic dye.
- Compound dye is used for staining of blood smear, e.g. Leishman's stain, Giemsa's stain and Wright's stain (Romanowsky stains).

iv. Amphoteric Dyes

These dyes are like compound dyes having both anionic and cationic groups, but both groups are present on the same ion. Such dyes can stain either the nucleus or the cytoplasm.

Leucocompound Dyes

- Leucocompound dye is one whose colour depends upon chromophoric groups.
- This chromophoric group can be reduced by addition of hydrogen atom at the double bond position. In a benzene ring, as a result of reduction, the dye loses its colour and becomes colourless—such a colourless dye is known as a leucocompound dye.
- These dyes are used for detection of oxidation–reduction reactions (Fig. 1.1).
- Both acidic and basic stains are used in microbiology and bacteriology in particular.
- The basic stains colour acidic constituents of cells such as nuclei and metachromatic granules more intensely than cytoplasmic material, which is stained by acidic stains.

AUXOPHORES

- Auxophores are necessary for the property of electrolytic dissociation, i.e. salt forming property.
- These are the binding groups (ionizable group) that allow binding to the object to be stained. Auxophores are of two types:
  1. **Acidic auxophores**—auxophores with hydroxyl group (OH)
  2. **Basic auxophores**—auxophores with the amino group (NH_2)

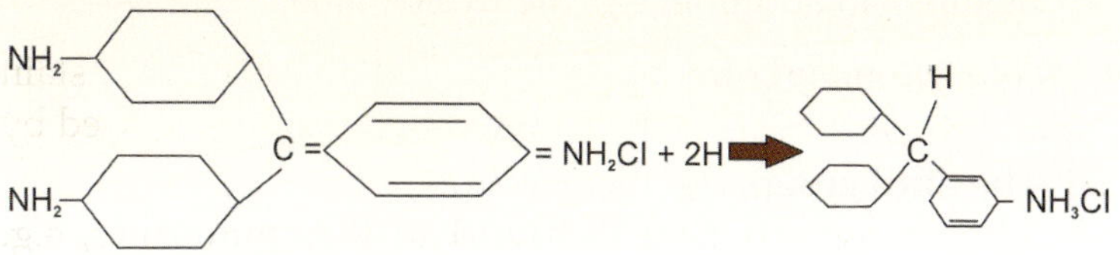

Fig.1.1: Reduction reaction in pararosaniline dye

- If OH groups are more in number in a compound dye, the dye is more acidic and if NH_2 groups are more in number then it is strongly basic.
- The NH_2 group is more strongly basic than the OH group is acidic (OH group is weakly acidic).
- If one OH and one NH_2 is present, the basic characteristic of the NH_2 predominates.
- Some dyes have the sulfonic group (SO_2OH) attached to benzene ring.
- The sulfonic group is a strongly acidic group possessing salt forming properties.

CHROMOPHORES

- Chromophores are groups that make organic compounds coloured.
- They are necessary for the property of colour.
- The dye must contain at least one chromophore that imparts the property of colour to the substance. Chromophores are of two types:
  1. Basic chromophores
  2. Acidic chromophores

1. Basic chromophores

These are of three types:

   i. **The azo group** is found in the azodyes, e.g. bismark brown, methyl red, methyl orange. These are derivatives of azobenzene.
  ii. **The azine group** is found in the phenazines, e.g. neutral red, safranine.
 iii. **The indamine group** is found in the indamines, the thiazines and other dyes. The thiazine shows the presence of sulfur in addition, e.g. methylene blue.

2. Acidic chromophores

These include:

   i. The nitro group, e.g. picric acid.
  ii. The quinonoid ring is found in the indamines, the xanthenes and the di- and triphenyl methanes, e.g. methyl violet, crystal violet, methyl green and pararosaniline.

CLASSIFICATION OF STAINS

- Both acidic and basic dyes used in microbiology and bacteriology in particular are classified based on the chromophoric groups present in them.
- The basic stains are the most important in bacteriology.

1. The Nitro Stains

These are acidic stains in which the chromophore is a nitro group (NO_2), e.g. picric acid and martius yellow.

2. The Azo Group

These are further subdivided into:

a. *Monoazo stains:* In these stains, the chromophore is a $-N = N-$ which joins together the benzene or naphthalene rings, e.g. methyl red, Sudan R, Sudan II.

b. *Diazo and polyazo stains:* In these stains, more than one chromophore ($-N = N-$) which joins together the benzene or naphthalene rings, e.g. Bismark brown, Sudan black, Evans blue, Sudan III, Sudan IV.

3. The Anthraquinone Group

These are stains in which the chromophore is a quinonoid ring and the chromogen is anthraquinone, e.g. alizarin and carmine.

4. The Thiazole Stains

These are stains containing thiazole ring in which the chromophore is a indamine group, e.g. titan yellow G.

5. The Quinonimine Stains

- These are stains in which there are two chromophores—the indamines group and the quinonoid ring.
- These are of following types:
  a. *The indamines*: Not important
  b. *The indophenols:* Not important
  c. *The thiazines:* These have a phenyl and a quininoid ring joined together by an atom of sulfur and one of nitrogen to form a third closed ring, e.g. methyl violet, methylene blue, methylene green, toluidine blue O, azure A and B.

   d. *The oxazines:* In these stains the sulfur of the thiazines is replaced by oxygen atom, e.g. crystal violet, resazurin.

   e. *The azines:* These are the derivatives of phenazines— containing two benzene rings or one benzene ring and one quinonoid ring joined together by two nitrogen atoms to form a third ring. These include—the aminoazines (e.g. neutral red, neutral violet), the safranines (e.g. safranine O, phenosafranine) and the indulines (e.g. nigrosine, induline).

6. Phenyl–Methane Stains

- These compounds are substituted methanes.
- One or more hydrogen atoms of methane may be replaced by methyl, ethyl or phenyl groups.
- The introduction of amino group and other groups, and substituted aminogroups result into large number of compounds.
- These include:
  - a. The diaminotriphenyl–methane stains, e.g. brilliant green, malachite green.
  - b. The triaminotriphenyl–methane stains, e.g. acid fuchsin, aniline blue, basic fuchsin, crystal violet, methyl violet, rosaniline, pararosaniline, methyl green, methyl blue.
  - c. The hydroxytriphenyl–methane stains, e.g. rosolic acid.
  - d. The diphenyl–naphthyl–methane stains, e.g. Victoria blue B, Victoria blue R, night blue.

7. The Xanthene Stains

- These are derivatives of xanthene.
- Some are basic and some are acidic.
- Commonly used as indicators.
- The examples are:
  - i. The pyronine stains
  - ii. The rhodamine stains
  - iii. The fluorane stains
  - iv. The phenolphthalein and the sulfonephthalein stains, e.g. bromocresol green, bromocresol purple, bromothymol

blue, cresol red, phenolphthalein, phenol red, thymol blue, etc.

v. *The acridine stains:* These are derivatives of acridine. Basically these are used as disinfectants against bacteria and protozoa, e.g. acridine orange, acridine yellow, acriflavine, atabrine, etc.

8. The Natural Stains

- These are stains which are extracted from natural sources.
- During early days, these were most commonly used stains.
- Now most of them are replaced by synthetic stains, which are reliable, cheaper and readily available.
- Only a few of them are important in bacteriology, e.g.
    i. *Indigo* obtained from plants of the genus *Indigofera.*
    ii. *Indigo carmine* having acidic property.
    iii. *Cochineal* obtained from insect–*Coccus cacti.*
    iv. *Carmine:* Cochineal + alum.
    v. *Orcein* obtained from *Lichens.*
    vi. Litmus obtained from *Lichens.*
    vii. *Brazilin* obtained from bane of Brazil wood.
    viii. *Haematoxylin* obtained from logwood—a legume growing in South America.

MORDANT, TRAPPING AGENT AND ACCENTUATOR

Mordant

- It is a substance that enhances the attraction between primary stain and cell cytoplasm, and helps to fix primary stain in the cell cytoplasm.
- The mordant forms insoluble compound with a stain and serves to fix the colour to the bacterial cell.
- The following are the examples of mordant:
    – Iodine
    – Tannic acid
    – Salts of aluminium
    – Iron
    – Tin

- Zinc
- Copper and chromium
- Aniline oil
- Phenol

• The mordant gives greater stability to the stain and it does not allow stain to be removed by water, alcohols or weak acids.
• Generally, mordant is applied first followed by the addition of staining solution or applied to the smear after primary stain, e.g. iodine applied after—crystal violet in Gram staining.
• In some staining procedures, the mordant is added to staining solution itself, e.g. phenol is mixed with basic fuchsin in acid fast staining.
• Staining of an organism without the use of mordant is called direct staining and staining with the use of mordant is known as indirect staining.

Trapping Agent

• It is different from mordant in that it is always applied after the stain.
• It forms large aggregates with the stain and causes precipitation of stain.
• The large precipitate is more difficult to remove from the stained object, e.g. iodine is used as a trapping agent to trap the primary stain in gram-positive bacteria.

Accentuator/Accelerator

• Accentuator is a chemical that may be added to a staining solution to speed up its reaction or to make its reaction more selective.
• Unlike mordant, accentuator does not combine with a stain, e.g. potassium hydroxide used in Loeffler's methylene blue acts as an accentuator and enhances staining power of staining solution.
• Staining of an organism without the use of mordant but using accentuator is called direct staining.
• It is also known as accelerator.

S.no.	Mordant	Accentuator
	Table 1.1: Differences between mordant and accentuator	
1.	Method of staining—indirect	Method of staining—direct
2.	Increase attraction between primary stain and cell cytoplasm	Speed up reaction
3.	Combine with stain	Does not combine with stain

Differences between mordant and accentuator are given in Table 1.1.

THEORIES OF STAINING

1. Physical Reaction

It is a reaction between two substances without the formation of a new compound. When bacteria are stained, there is no evidence that the stain has been changed chemically to form a new compound. The stain can be extracted from cells by long immersion in water, alcohol or other solvent. The factors that play an important role in physical reaction are capillarity, osmosis, adsorption and absorption.

2. Chemical Reaction

According to this theory, some parts of the cell/tissue are acidic in nature/character, e.g. nuclei of the cells, whereas other parts of the cell/tissue are basic in nature/character, e.g. cytoplasm. The synthetic stains are either anionic (acidic) or cationic (basic). According to this theory the acidic constituents of the cell/tissue (nucleus) have an affinity for basic stains and react with basic stains, and the basic constituents of the cell/tissue (cytoplasm) have an affinity for acidic stains and react with acidic stains. This interaction results into formation of a new compound.

MICROBIOLOGICAL USES OF STAINS

The microbiological uses of stains include:

1. *Staining of microbes:* Bacteria, yeasts, fungi, and protozoa in dried smears or in tissues.
2. *Use as indicators:* Incorporated in culture media as an indicator to indicate the presence of a particular bacterium.

3. *Use as selective agent because of their selective inhibitory action:* They can be incorporated in culture media as selective agent, e.g. malachite green is incorporated in Lowenstein-Jensen medium, crystal violet in Pike's medium, etc.

4. Bacteriological stains—used to study bacterial cytology.

PREPARATION AND STORAGE OF STAINING SOLUTIONS

Preparation of Stains

- The powder form of stain is weighed accurately.
- The weighed powder is ground in a mortar with diluents—add a small amount of diluents to start with and go on adding the diluents slowly till the required quantity of diluents is added.
- The staining solution prepared so is to be filtered before use.
- The storing bottles are to be labeled properly with details of concentration of staining reagent and date of preparation.

Storage of Stains

- Proper care should be exercised in storage of staining reagents.
- Staining reagent should be stored in well-closed glass Stoppard bottles (except for Loeffler's methylene blue).
- Staining reagents should be stored in dark and cool place and out of direct sunlight.
- For frequent use, flexible plastic or glass dropping bottles can be used. These bottles are to be cleaned thoroughly before refilling.
- Staining reagent should not be stored in the close proximity of the acids and ammonia.
- Distilled water used for preparation of staining reagents should be freshly prepared and neutral in nature.

2

Types of Staining

There are two important types of staining techniques:

VITAL STAINING

- The staining techniques in which microorganisms are not killed.
- Vital staining is a study of microbes, bacteria in particular, in living condition after imparting colour to microbes.
- Examples of vital staining are:
  - Use of diluted methylene blue, crystal violet and haematoxylin for the study of parasites in living conditions.
  - Use of 1:5000 dilution of methylene blue for the study of microfilaria (Sharp, 1927).
  - Use of 1:1000 and 1:10,000 dilutions of methylene blue and crystal violet to study bacteria in living conditions. These staining solutions have been reported to be suitable for the rapid and accurate study of bacterial motility. Particularly crystal violet at 1: 1000 to 1: 10, 000 dilutions gives very good results (Nagoba et al., 1991).

SUPRAVITAL STAINING

- The staining techniques in which microorganisms are killed.
- Supravital staining methods are further classified into the following types:
  - i. Simple staining
  - ii. Negative staining
  - iii. Impregnation staining

     iv. Differential staining
     v. Special staining

i. Simple Staining

- It is also known as monochrome staining (*mono* means single and *chrome* means colouring agent)
- It uses watery solution of only one simple basic dye, e.g. methylene blue, methyl violet, crystal violet or carbol fuchsin.
- It provides the colour contrast but imparts same colour to all microbes in the smear.

ii. Negative Staining (Background Staining)

- In this method, a staining solution provides an uniformly coloured background against which the unstained bacteria stand out in contrast.
- In this, the background is stained and organisms appear as colourless objects against a dark background.
- This method is used for demonstration of capsule and spirochaetes.
- It can also be used for the study of bacterial motility.

iii. Impregnation Staining

- Organisms, which are very thin to be seen under light microscope, are rendered visible by increasing their thickness by impregnating silver on their surface.
- This method is used for demonstration of organisms like spirochaetes and bacterial flagella.

iv. Differential Staining

- The staining methods, which differentiate two types of organisms, are known as differential staining.
- They impart different colours to different bacteria or bacterial structures, e.g. Gram stain and acid-fast stain.

v. Special Staining

- The staining methods used for demonstration of specific surface structures like capsules and flagella and as well as internal structures like endospores, which are difficult to reveal by conventional staining techniques, are known as special staining.

- The purpose is to specifically enhance these structures.

OTHER TYPES OF STAINING

Other staining methods/techniques used in microbiology include:

i. Progressive Staining

- A staining method/technique in which stain is applied to the section until the desired intensity of colour is reached or attained.
- The tissue is left in the staining solution till it retains the desired amount of colouration.
- In progressive staining, once the stain is taken up by the tissue it is not removed.
- Differentiation in progressive staining relies solely on the selective affinity of stains for different tissue elements.

ii. Regressive Staining

- A staining method/technique in which tissues are over stained and excess stain is then removed selectively until the desired intensity is obtained.
- In a regressive stain, the tissue is first over stained and then partially decolourized.
- Differentiation is usually controlled visually by examination with a microscope.
- When regressive staining is employed, a sharper degree of differentiation is obtained than with progressive staining.

iii. Specific Staining

A staining method/technique in which staining reagent used acts only on certain constituents of the cells and tissues and have a little or no effect on other constituents.

iv. Metachromatic Staining

- A staining method/technique in which staining reagents used stain the constituents of the cells and tissues in various shades of their own fundamental colour.
- The staining reagent has the capacity to stain different elements of a cell or tissue in different colours or shades.
- In a phenomenon of metachromasia, a staining reagent with a particular colour stains a cell component by giving it different colour than its original colour.
- This colour shift is called metachromasia.
- Many stains show this phenomenon but the thiazine group (e.g. toluidine blue) stains are good for this type of staining.

v. Bipolar Staining

- A staining method/technique in which the two ends of cells are more deeply coloured/stained than the center part of the cells, e.g. the plague bacilli (*Yersinia pestis*) show bipolar staining.
- A bipolar stain is a particular staining pattern that colors only the two opposite poles of the microorganism, leaving the rest of the part unstained or of a lighter color.

vi. Beaded Staining

- A simple staining method/technique in which staining reagent used does not stain bacterial cells evenly, e.g. diphtheria bacilli (*Corynebacterium diphtheriae*) show alternate dark and light bars known as beaded appearance.
- Beaded appearance is also seen in *Mycobacterium tuberculosis*.

3

Smear Preparation

A smear is a thin uniform film of a material made on a glass slide or cover slip.

METHODS OF MAKING FILM/SMEAR PREPARATION

Film/smear is prepared either on glass slide or cover slip. Glass slides are commonly used for smear preparation.

Dimensions of the Slide

- Size—76 mm × 26 mm × 1.15 mm.
- Refractive index 1.53 ± 0.02

Dimensions of the Cover Slip

Size—preferably 20 mm × 20 mm, however 22 mm × 22 mm with thickness 0.1 mm (No. 1) can also be used.

Cleaning of Slides and Cover Slips

Cleaning of Slides

- Wipe the slide with a clean dry cotton cloth and then holding its end with forceps, roast it grease-free by passing it 6–12 times through a blue Bunsen flame or moist the finger with water, rub it on the surface of soap and then smear the surface of the slide then clean with a clean cloth.
- For special purposes, slides are to be cleaned by immersion in concentrated H_2SO_4 saturated with potassium dichromate for several days at room temperature. If the slide is perfectly clean, a drop of water can spread over its surface in a thin even film; otherwise water collects into small drops and a film cannot be made.

- Like glass slides, cover slips are cleaned by dichromate—sulfuric acid solution, then washed with tap water and then with distilled water, and are stored in a stopper jar in a 50% alcohol. Before use, they are dried using clean cloth. For routine use, the cover slips are used directly after removal of grit and dust with the help of a clean cloth.

Labeling of the Slides

- Every slide should be labeled clearly with date, number and patient's name or specimen number on the opposite side of the smear.
- A smear/film area should also be marked.
- A special pencil (diamond or grease pencil) or special marking pen should be used as ordinary pencil/pen marks are washed out during staining process.

Making Films/Smears

- In case of fluid materials such as broth culture, or specimens of urine, sputum, pus, or other body fluids, one loopful or more is taken with the help of inoculating loop and then spread thinly on the slide. The film is allowed to dry and then fixed by passing the dried smear for three times slowly through the flame.
- In case of purulent specimen—purulent material is spread thinly using a sterile wire loop.
- In case of nonpurulent fluid—the fluid is centrifuged and smear is prepared from a drop of sediment.
- In case of sputum—a clean stick is used to transfer and spread the purulent and caseous material on slide.
- In case of swab—a swab is rolled on slide. This is important, when smear is observed for intracellular microbes like *Neisseria*. The rolling of swab avoids damage to pus cells.
- In case of solid material, such as cultures on agar, a loopful of normal saline or clean water is placed on the glass slide. The inoculation loop is then sterilized and a minute quantity of material obtained from colony by just touching the growth is transferred to the drop on the glass slide and thoroughly

emulsified. The mixture is then spread evenly on the slide. The resulting film/smear is then dried and fixed as above.

- In case of very tiny colonies that might be lost in even a small drop of saline, a sterile wooden applicator stick can be used to touch the colony and obtain a bit of growth. This material is then rubbed directly onto the slide, where it can be easily stained.

Ideal Smear

- Smear should not be too thin or too thick.
- It should be spread evenly covering an area of about 15–20 mm diameter and thin enough so that the newspaper letters are just visible through the smear.

PREPARATION OF BLOOD SMEARS FOR EXAMINATION OF BLOOD PARASITES

- Examination of blood smears forms an important part in accurate identification of parasites in blood—haemoparasites.
- Two types of blood smears/films are generally used. These are:
  - i. Thin blood smears/films
  - ii. Thick blood smears/films

i. Thin Blood Smears/Films

- These are of monolayer thickness.
- These films allow specific identification of species—used primarily for identification purpose.
- Disadvantage of thin blood film—as it allows the examination of less amount of blood, the number of parasites per field are less as compared to the thick blood smear.

Preparation of Thin Blood Smear

- For smear preparation use an alcohol cleaned and grease free slide. If old slides are to be used, first clean them with detergent and then with 70% ethyl alcohol.
- Place a small drop of fresh blood on a clean slide, about 1.5 cm from the end of the slide.

- Touch the drop of blood with the edge of another slide and allow the blood to spread along the edge.
- Quickly push the second slide or the spreader across at about a 30° angle, along the surface of the horizontal slide to the far end.
- This helps in uniform distribution of blood and to form a thin smear/film.
- Allow the thin blood film to dry, and then stain the smear with Romanowsky stain.

ii. Thick Blood Smears/Films

- These are several layers thick and are primarily used as a screening procedure.
- These are more sensitive method for detection of parasites as compared to thin smears, because they allow examination of large amount of blood.
- Disadvantage of thick blood smear—species identification of parasites cannot be made.

Preparation of Thick Blood Smear

- Place two or three small drops of fresh blood (without any anticoagulant) on a grease-free alcohol cleaned slide.
- With the help of the corner of another slide, spread and mix the drops of blood over an area of about 2 cm in diameter.
- The mixing is continued for about 30 seconds to prevent formation of any fibrin strands which may conceal the parasites in a stained smear. If blood containing anticoagulant is used, 2 or 3 drops may be spread over an area of about 1 cm in diameter.
- Allow the thick blood film to air dry at room temperature.
- After the smear is dried in air, lyse the thick blood film with distilled water for dehaemoglobinisation.
- After the dehaemoglobinisation of smear, stain it with Romanowsky stain.

Combined Thick and Thin Smears/Films

- The thick and thin smears/films can be prepared on the same slide.

- This type of smears may be helpful in field surveys.
- Sufficient time should be allowed for the thick portion of the smear to dry before staining.
- Both the thick and thin blood films should be stained simultaneously.

Fixation of the Smear

- After preparation of smear, it needs to be fixed to preserve microorganisms and to prevent smears being washed from slides during staining.
- After smear is prepared, it is allowed to air dry thoroughly. Heating of the smear without allowing it to air dry may result in formation of air bubbles during heating and may result into the formation of artifacts. Hence, the smear is air-dried and then it can be fixed by the following methods.

1. Physical Method

- *For example:* Heat fixation: The smear is fixed by passing the dried slide film for three times slowly through the flame or by heating the slide, i.e. by holding the slide over flame for few seconds with smear upwards. Overheating of slide should be avoided as it distorts the cells.
- Heat coagulates the protein content of the bacterial cell wall and thus, helps in fixation.
- Heating fixes the smear to the slide and prevents the washing away of the smear material.
- Heat fixation can damage microorganisms and alter their staining characters, if excessive heat is used.
- Heat fixation damages leukocytes and is therefore unsuitable for fixing smears which may contain intracellular organisms like *N. gonorrhoeae* and *N. meningitidis*.
- *M. tuberculosis* from sputum smears are not killed by usual heat fixation method.
- The heat fixation is recommended for *M. leprae* smears.

2. Chemical Methods

Alcohol fixation: This method is far less damaging to microorganisms than heat. Usually used to fix blood smears.

i. *Absolute methanol or ethanol:* Leukocytes/pus cells are well preserved and hence, recommended for fixing smears of Gram-negative diplococci, which are intracellular in nature.

ii. *70% v/v methanol or ethanol: M. tuberculosis* are rapidly killed in sputum smears after applying 70% v/v alcohol.

Other Chemical Fixatives

- It is sometimes necessary to fix smears containing dangerous microorganisms, the purpose is to ensure all the microorganisms are killed. For example: 40 g/L potassium permanganate is recommended for smears which may contain anthrax bacilli.
- Formaldehyde vapours are sometimes recommended for fixing smears which may contain *Mycobacterium* species.
- Chemical fixatives are used for fixation of infectious tissue.
- Other chemicals used for fixation are formalin, mercuric chloride, osmic acid, etc.

Preparation of Tissue Sections

The following steps are involved in preparation of tissue sections.

i. *Fixation of Tissue*

- For fixation, small pieces of tissue are to be used.
- Tissue must be fixed by using a large amount of fixing fluid.
- The appropriate fixing fluid must be employed, e.g.
  - *Formalin (10%) is commonly used:* It is a good general fixative. It possesses all the qualities of good fixatives. It is not good where fine details are to be observed, e.g. for examination of material containing protozoa.
  - *Schaudinn's fluid:* Containing absolute ethyl alcohol and saturated aqueous solution of mercuric chloride is used for protozoa.
  - *Bouin's fluid:* Containing saturated aqueous solution of picric acid, formalin and glacial acetic acid is used for the viral inclusion bodies.
  - *Other fixatives* include: Susa fixative and Flemming's fluid.

ii. *Embedding of Tissue*

- Paraffin sections are most commonly used.
- Before the tissue is fixed in paraffin, all water must be removed from the tissue material and to be replaced by a fluid with which melted paraffin wax mixes well. This is necessary for proper embedding of the tissue.
- Water is first removed with several changes of alcohol.
- The alcohol is replaced by fluid such as xylene, acetone or chloroform—a fluid which is solvent for both alcohol and paraffin wax.
- After the water is removed, the tissue is finally embedded in paraffin wax.
- The procedure of embedding is as follows:
    - After fixation of tissue, small pieces of tissue are placed in 90% alcohol for 2–5 hours.
    - Transferred to absolute alcohol for 2 hours.
    - The process of dehydration is completed in absolute alcohol for 2 hours.
    - Transferred to a mixture of absolute alcohol and chloroform (equal parts) till the tissue sinks or overnight.
    - Placed in pure chloroform for 6 hours.
    - Transferred to a mixture of equal parts of chloroform and paraffin wax and kept in a melted state in the paraffin oven.
    - Placed in a pure melted paraffin in the oven at 55°C for 2 hours, preferably in a vacuum embedding oven.
    - The tissue embedded in blocks of paraffin is used for section cutting.

iii. *Section Cutting*

- The tissue embedded in blocks of paraffin are cut out, trimmed and sections of 5 µm thick are cut by means of a microtome.
- The sections are flattened on warm water, floated onto slides and allowed to dry.

iv. *Staining of Tissue Section*

- For better penetration of watery stain, it is necessary to remove the paraffin from the section.
- The paraffin is first removed with xylene, the xylene is then removed with alcohol (95% ethanol) and the alcohol is replaced with water. For this, the slide with the paraffin section is placed in a jar of xylene for a few minutes to remove the paraffin. The section is then treated with a few drops of absolute alcohol, when it immediately becomes opaque. A few drops of 50% alcohol are poured on, and the slide is finally washed in water. If the tissue is fixed in a fixative containing mercuric chloride (e.g. Zenker's fluid), the section should be treated with Gram's iodine solution for a few minutes, then with 95% alcohol and finally with water.
- The section is then stained by the appropriate staining method.
- After staining and washing with water, the slide is wiped all round with a clean cloth to remove excess water. The bulk of the water in the section may be removed by pressing between fluffless blotting paper.
- The section is dehydrated by treating immediately with a few drops of 95% alcohol and then with absolute alcohol and cleared in xylene by immersing in it. When the bacteria are readily decolourized with alcohol, aniline-xylene (aniline, 2 parts: xylene, 1 part) should be used for dehydration.
- When cleared, the slide is removed, and excess xylene round the section is wiped away.

v. *Mounting of Section*

- Mounted in Canada balsam—a drop of Canada balsam is applied and the section is mounted under a no. 1 cover slip.
- Alternatively, DPX (consists of polystyrene—a synthetic resin dissolved in xylol, with a plasticizer—dibutyl phthalate) can be used for mounting instead of Canada balsam. DPX medium is water—clear, inert and does not become acid or cause fading of stained preparations. It is used in the same way as Canada balsam.

Discarding of Slides

- After the films/smears have been prepared and examined, the slides should be discarded into a pot containing one percent hypochlorite solution.
- They should not be cleaned and reused. As it is difficult to ensure that all the microorganisms are removed from the smear.

4

Simple Staining
(Monochrome Staining)

- A staining method/technique in which a watery solution of simple basic dye is used, e.g. methylene blue, dilute carbol fuchsin, methyl violet, crystal violet. Sometimes, a watery solution of basic dye is used along with mordant to allow better penetration. These dyes provide the colour contrast but impart same colour to all microbes in the smear.
- Simple staining is also known as monochrome staining (*mono* means one/single and *chrome* means colour) as the object is stained with only one/single watery solution of a simple basic dye in one application.

STAINING REAGENTS

Following staining reagents are used for simple staining:

1. *Loeffler's methylene blue:* The composition of this is saturated solution of methylene blue in alcohol—300 ml KOH, 0.01% in distilled water—1000 ml
   - Add potassium hydroxide to distilled water
   - Add saturated alcoholic solution of methylene blue
   - Filter through filter paper after 24 h.

2. *Polychrome methylene blue:* This is prepared by allowing Loeffler's methylene blue to 'ripen' slowly. There are two methods of ripening:
   i. *Slow method of ripening:* In this method, the stain is kept in bottles, which are half filled and shaken at intervals to aerate thoroughly the contents. This slow process of oxidation of methylene blue forms a violet-coloured compound that gives the stain its polychrome property. It takes 12 months or more to complete the process of ripening.

ii. *Quick method of ripening:* In this method, the stain may be ripened quickly by adding 1% potassium carbonate (K_2CO_3) to Loeffler's methylene blue

This preparation is useful in a manner similar to Loeffler's methylene blue.

3. *Dilute carbol fuchsin:* Prepared by diluting carbol fuchsin used in Ziehl-Neelsen stain for 10–20 times with water. It is useful for staining *Borrelia* spp.

Specimens

Pus, cerebrospinal fluid and various aspirates.

STAINING PROCEDURE

Steps of staining procedures in simple staining are:
- Prepare smear and fix it by heating gently in a Bunsen flame. Chemical fixatives such as formalin, mercuric chloride, methyl alcohol or osmic acid are used for sections of infected tissues and infected blood smears.
- Stain the heat fixed smear by flooding it with one of the staining solutions and allowing it to remain covered with the stain for the time designated below:
  - Methylene blue: 2–3 minutes
  - Carbol fuchsin: 10–25 seconds
  - Crystal violet: 30 seconds
- Over-staining with carbol fuchsin must be avoided as this is an intense stain.
- Pour off staining solution
- Wash with water
- Allow it to air dry/blot dry-wipe the back of the slide and blot the stained surface with bibulous paper or with a paper towel.
- Observe under oil immersion lens (100X).

Observations (Figs 4.1 and 4.2)
- Bacteria appear blue/violet/pink depending on staining soloution used
- Background—colourless

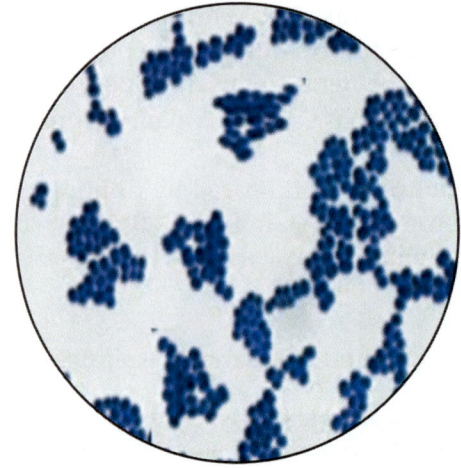

Fig. 4.1: Cocci stained with methylene blue

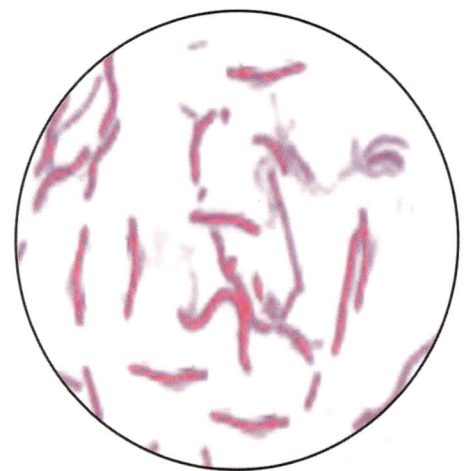

Fig. 4.2: Bacilli stained with dilute carbol fuchsin

Uses

The simple stain can be used to determine cell shape, size and arrangement.

1. *Loeffler's methylene blue:* Most useful to demonstrate the characteristic morphology of polymorphs, lymphocytes and

other cells more clearly than stronger stains such as Gram's stain or dilute carbol fuchsin. It is also useful for staining *Yersinia pestis* (safety pin appearance) and leukocytes in faecal preparations (Fig. 4.3).

2. *Polychrome methylene blue:* It is used in a manner similar to Loeffler's methylene blue and also used to stain the capsules of *Bacillus anthracis* (McFadyean's reaction).

3. *Dilute carbol fuchsin:* It is used for demonstration of *Borrelia* spp.

Mechanism

- The surface of bacterial cells is acidic in nature. The overall nature of bacterial cell surface is acidic in nature because of carboxyl group located on the cell surface due to acidic amino acids. When ionization of carboxyl group takes place, it gives negative charge to the cell surface:

$$COOH \rightarrow COO^- + H^+$$

- This negatively charged ion combines firmly with coloured positively charged ion of the basic dye. The result is bond formation between the stain and cell component/surface that finally leads to staining of cells. The stain is retained through

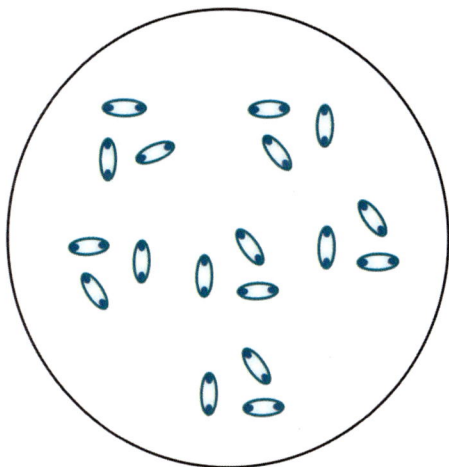

Fig. 4.3: *Yersinia pestis*—safety pin appearance stained with Loeffler's methylene blue

subsequent washing with water and the excess of the stain is removed.

- Simple stain not only shows the presence of microorganisms but also shows the nature of the cellular content in exudates.
- Acidic dyes having coloured anion do not stain bacteria strongly except at very high acidic pH and these can be used for negative staining. Cells or structures that stain with basic dyes at normal pH are basophilic and those that stain with acidic stains are acidophilic.

5

Negative Staining

- Negative staining, also known as background staining, is a technique in which microorganisms are not stained but are made visible against dark background.
- In this, the background is stained and organisms appear as colourless and refractile objects against a dark background.
- It is also known as indirect staining.
- This method is used for demonstration of capsule and spirochaetes.
- Its use has also been reported for the study of bacterial motility.

STAINING REAGENTS

Acidic dyes such as India Ink, nigrosin or eosin is used.

1. India Ink

- Pelikan Drawin ink, 17 Black (India Ink) containing 0.3% tricresol as a preservative is recommended.
- It must be dense, homogenous and finely granular.
- As India ink may be contaminated with capsulated or non-capsulated microorganisms, hence, it is necessary to examine microscopically each bottle to rule out microbial contamination.
- If it is contaminated, the bottle should not be used.
- A modification of India ink using 2% mercurochrome is used for demonstration of the capsulated budding yeast cells of *Cryptococcus neoformans*. The use of 2% mercurochrome increases the clearity.

31

2. Nigrosin

- Nigrosin is prepared as follows:

  Nigrosin   10 g

  Warm distilled water   100 ml

  (Alternatively, boil for 30 minutes in an Erlenmeyer flask, when warm distilled water is not used).

  Formalin (40%)   0.5 ml

- Formalin is added as a preservative. The reagent prepared so is filtered twice through double filter.

3. Eosin

One percent aqueous solution is prepared

Eosin   1 gm

Distilled water   100 ml

STAINING PROCEDURES

- Clean the slide using suitable cleaning material. Gently dry the slide with a lint-free cloth (alternatively, commercially available pre-cleaned slides can be used).
- Place a small drop (one or two loopful) of the negative stain (India ink) near the end of the slide.
- Transfer one loopful of the culture or other material containing microbes to the India ink (used in Bussis India ink method) or nigrosin solution (used in Fleming's nigrosin method) and mix them properly.
- With the help of another slide, the thin film is made from the drop, i.e. by holding a clean slide at about a 20° angle to the first slide; touch the edge of the clean slide to the drop so that the mixture spreads across the edge and then spread the suspension across the surface of the slide by drawing the clean slide away from the mixture.
- Allow smear to air dry—do not heat fix.
- Observe smear under the oil immersion objective (100X) of bright field microscope.
- Record the findings.

Observations

- In Bussis India ink method
  - Bacteria: Clear transparent objects
  - Background: Brown
- In Fleming's nigrosin method
  - Bacteria: Bright unstained objects
  - Background: Dark
  - In Fleming's nigrosin method: Some bacilli, e.g. belonging to coliform and *Haemophilus* group show a slightly dark patch in the central portion that looks like a nucleus.

WET INDIA INK FILMS FOR CAPSULES

- Clean the slide using suitable cleaning material and wipe it carefully to make it free from particle of dust or girt.
- Place a large loopful of undiluted India Ink on the slide.
- Emulsify a very small portion of solid bacterial culture or a small loopful of liquid culture in the India Ink or
- Rub the speck of solid material on the slide surface just besides the ink before mixing it into the ink.
- Place a clean, girt-free cover slip on the ink drop and press it down through a sheet of blotting paper so that the film becomes very thin and thus pale in colour. The film should be so thin that the bacterial cell with its capsule is gripped between the slide and cover slip.
- If the film is left too thick, the capsule is obscured by the overlying ink. If it is pressed too thin, the capsules are crushed or flatten and the ink background becomes too pale to give a good contrast.
- Observe under the oil immersion objective (100X).

Observations

- Microscopic examination under the oil immersion objective shows—the highly refractile outline of the bacterium.
- The clear space between this refractile surface membrane and the dark background of the ink particles, there is a capsule—the capsular zone may be from a fraction of micrometer to several micrometers in width.

- This clear zone is not seen in noncapsulated bacteria.
- When slime layer is present as in solid bacterial culture, it can be seen as irregular masses of amorphous material.
- Loose slime is generally invisible if the preparations are made from the culture in liquid medium.

Advantage

As there is no drying or fixation of smear, there is no shrinkage of capsule.

Special Recommendations

It is recommended that wet India ink films should be examined with a phase contrast microscope. Since the bodies of the bacteria are not stained in such films, their outlines are only faintly visible under the ordinary microscope. With the phase contrast microscope, the bodies of bacteria appear dark and are seen in clear contrast to the bright capsular zones surrounding them.

DRY INDIA INK FILMS FOR CAPSULES

- Place a loopful of 6% of glucose in water at one end of a slide.
- Add a small amount of bacterial culture to this and mix to form an even suspension.
- Add a loopful of India ink to the drop and mix it.
- Spread the mixture over the slide in the form of a thin film with the edge of second glass slide.
- Allow it to air dry.
- Fix the smear by pouring over it some undiluted Leishman stain or methyl alcohol.
- Drain off excess at once and dry thoroughly by warming over a flame.
- Drop on methyl violet solution as used in Gram's stain and stain for 1–2 minutes.
- Wash in water.
- Blot and dry.
- Observe smear under the oil immersion objective (100X).

Observations

- Bacteria are stained darkly with violet dye
- Capsule appears as a clear zone between bacterium and the dark ink background.

EOSIN FOR WET FILMS

- Eosin can be used for negative staining of intestinal parasites.
- Wet film of stool is a standard preparation prepared by emulsifying small quantity of faeces in a drop of saline on a glass slide and applying cover slip on it avoiding air bubbles.
- Instead of a drop of saline, a drop of eosin used for staining wet films.
- The eosin wet film is observed under low and high power objectives.

Observations

- Trophozoites and cysts of protozoa, and larvae and eggs of helminthes appear pearly white objects
- Background: Pink
- Eosin also indicates viability of cysts—live cysts appear unstained and dead cysts appear pink in colour.

NEGATIVE STAIN FOR BACTERIAL MOTILITY

- One ml of specimen or one ml of peptone water culture is mixed with one ml of nigrosin (1:10 to 1:1000 dilution of nigrosin can be used).
- A loopful of this mixture is taken on cover slip and inverted as in hanging drop preparation method.
- This preparation is observed under low power objective (10X) to adjust edge and finally under high power objective (40X) to observe motility.

Observations

- Motile bacteria are unstained
- Background is dark
  Motile bacteria are readily seen against the dark background.

Advantages

Detection of motility is rapid and more accurate as compared to routine hanging drop preparation.

Uses of Negative Staining

- India ink or 10% nigrosin is used for demonstration of capsules of microorganisms like *Streptococcus pneumoniae, Klebsiella pneumoniae,* Group B streptococci, Group D streptococci, *Haemophilus influenzae* and *Cryptococcus neoformans.*
- Spirochaetes can be viewed by using India ink.
- Used for demonstration of bacterial motility.
- Eosin is used for demonstration of parasitic elements in stool.

Mechanism

Two different explanations have been proposed (Figs 5.1 and 5.2):

1. Negative stains (acidic stains) having negative charges do not combine with negatively charged particles on bacterial cell surface. On the other hand they settle around outer boundary and form deposit around the cell that results into appearance of dark background against which bacteria are seen colourless.

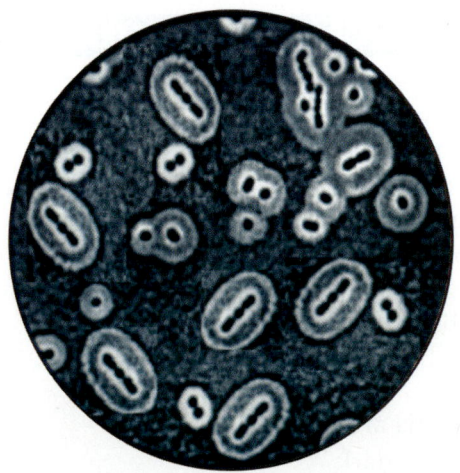

Fig. 5.1: Negative stain showing bacterial capsule

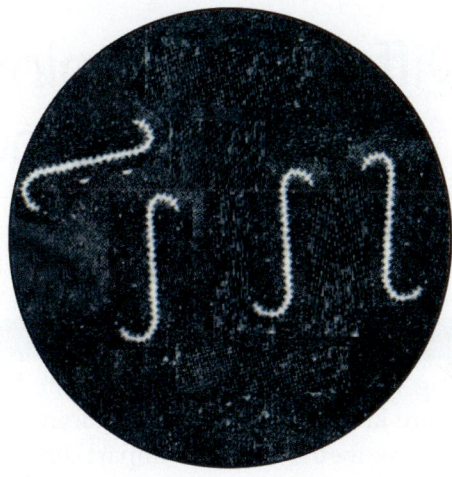

Fig. 5.2: Negative stain showing spirochaetes

2. Negative stains have acidic pH and cell cytoplasm is also acidic in nature, hence there is no attraction between acidic stain and acidic cytoplasm and that is why the bacterial body is not stained.

6

Differential Staining I: Gram Staining

DEFINITION

- The staining methods, which differentiate two types of organisms, are known as differential staining.
- In these staining methods, stains impart different colour to different bacteria or bacterial structures, e.g. Gram staining, acid-fast staining, Leishman's staining, Giemsa staining, etc.
- These staining methods use two different coloured stains/dyes, called as primary stain and counter stain to differentiate/separate/distinguish cell types or parts.

GRAM STAINING

- It is a differential staining method, which differentiates bacterial species into two large groups—Gram-positive and Gram-negative, based on the chemical and physical properties of their cell walls.
- Gram staining method divides bacteria based on whether or not they resist decolourization with alcohol or acetone after staining with primary stain and subsequent application of mordant.
- Gram-positive bacteria resist decolourization and remain stained as a dark purple in colour while the Gram-negative bacteria are decolourized and are then counter stained light pink/red in colour by the subsequent application of counter stain.
- It is named after the Hans Christian Gram (1853-1938) who originally devised it in 1882 (but published in 1884).
- It is one of the most widely used staining methods in bacteriology for identification of bacteria.

HISTORY

- It is a staining method devised by the histologist **Christian Gram** (1884) to stain bacteria in tissue. Gram used aniline gentian violet as primary stain, Lugol's iodine as a mordant, absolute alcohol as a decolourizer and bismark brown as a counter stain.
- This original method of Gram is modified by Burke (1922), Kopeloff and Beerman (1922), Jensen, Weigert and Preston and Morrell (1962).

Staining Reagents

Gram stain uses four reagents

1. *Primary stain (crystal violet, methyl violet or gentian violet)*

Crystal violet or methyl violet	5 gm
Distilled water	1000 ml

   Filter before use

2. *Mordant:* Mordant used is Gram's or Lugol's iodine.
   - **Gram's iodine**

Iodine	10 gm
Potassium iodide	20 gm
Distilled water	1000 ml

     Dissolve 20 gm potassium iodide in 250 ml of distilled water and then add 10 gm iodine; when dissolved make up to 1000 ml with distilled water.
   - **Lugol's iodine**

Iodine	10 gm
Potassium iodide	20 gm
Distilled water	300 ml

     Prepare as above and store. Dilute this for five times with distilled water before use.

3. *Decolourizer*

   Absolute alcohol (ethyl alcohol), acetone or ethanol–acetone mixture can be used as decolourizers.

4. *Counter stain*
   - **Safranine**

Safranine	2 gm
Distilled water	100 ml

- **Neutral red**

Neutral red	1 gm
1% acetic acid	2 ml
Distilled water	1000 ml

Procedure

Routine Procedure of Gram staining

- Prepare smear from clinical specimen, culture smear of csolony or broth culture on a clean glass slide, allow it to air dry and fix it by flaming. If the smear is for detection of *Neisseria* spp., it is to be fixed with methanol for two minutes.
- **Primary staining:** Cover smear with a few drops of pararosaline dye such as crystal violet, methyl violet or gentian violet and allow it to act for 30–60 seconds—this primary stain renders all the bacteria uniformly violet.
- **Application of mordant:** Pour off the primary stain and apply Gram's iodine. Allow it to act for 1–2 minutes and wash with water - this results in formation of a dye-iodine complex in the cytoplasm. The slide is again washed in water.
- **Decolourization:** Decolourize the smear with an organic solvent—for decolourization of smear keep the slide in tilted position and apply decolourizer (absolute alcohol or acetone) drop by drop for 10–30 seconds or until the colour oozes from slide. A mixture of acetone–ethyl alcohol (1:1) can also be used for decolourization. The process of decolourization is fairly quick and should not exceed 30 seconds for thin smears. Acetone is a potent decolourizer and when used alone can decolourize the smear in 2–3 seconds. A mixture of ethanol and acetone acts more slowly than pure acetone. Decolourization is the most crucial part of Gram staining and errors can occur here. Prolonged decolourization can lead to over-decolourized smear and a very short decolourization period may lead to under-decolourized smear. After the smear is decolorized, it is washed in water without any delay.
- **Counter staining:** Counter stain with a stain of contrasting colour—the smear is finally treated with a few drops of safranin, carbol fuchsin or neutral red for 15–30 seconds.

- Wash with water and blot dry.
- Observe the slide under 100X after putting a drop of cedarwood oil.

Observations

- Gram-positive bacteria are seen as violet-coloured whereas Gram-negative bacteria are seen as red pink-coloured.
- Gram stain divides bacteria in two broad groups as follows:
  - **Gram-positive bacteria**—these bacteria resist decolourization and retain the colour of the primary stain and appear violet.

Examples

- Gram-positive cocci—pneumococci, streptococci and staphylococci (Fig. 6.1).
- Gram-positive bacilli—clostridia, corynebacteria and *Bacillus* spp (Fig. 6.2).
  - Gram-negative bacteria—these bacteria are decolourized by alcohol and therefore, take counter stain and appear red.

Examples

- Gram-negative cocci—gonococci and meningococci (Fig. 6.3).

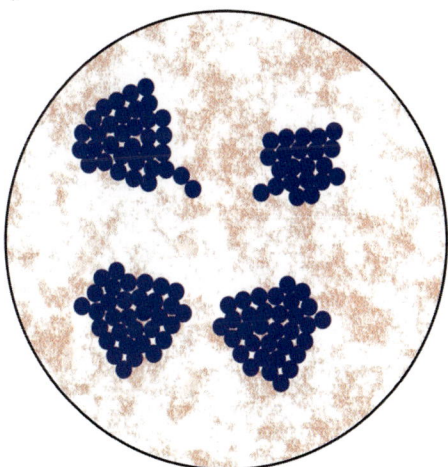

Fig. 6.1: Gram-positive cocci

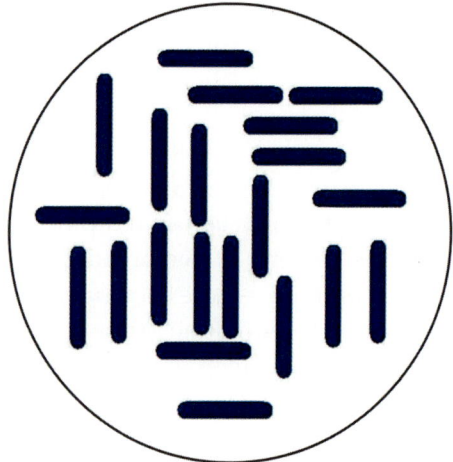

Fig. 6.2: Gram-positive bacilli

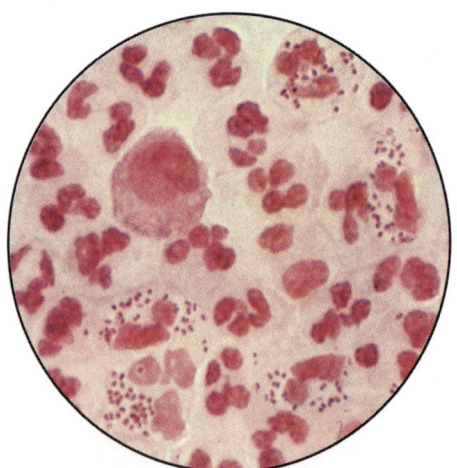

Fig. 6.3: Gram-negative cocci

- Gram-negative bacilli—*E. coli, Salmonella, Shigella, V. cholerae,* etc. (Fig. 6.4).
- Background/pus cells/epithelial cells and their nuclei appear red in colour while the fibrin in a clinical specimen may appear Gram-positive.

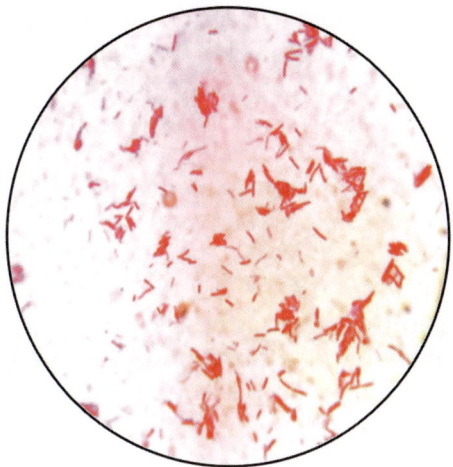

Fig. 6.4: Gram-negative bacilli

Control Smears

In order to ascertain whether the staining procedure is satisfactorily conducted or not, a control smear of known Gram-positive organism (e.g. *Staph. aureus*) and a known Gram-negative organism (e.g. *E. coli*) must be stained simultaneously.

2. Procedure for Staining of Sections

The steps are as follows:
- Remove paraffin with xylol or benzol
- Treat the section with absolute alcohol (100% ethanol) and wash with tap water
- Cover the smear with methyl violet and allow it to act for 5 minutes
- Wash off stain with an excess of iodine solution, cover smear with iodine and allow it to act for 2 minutes
- Decolourize smear with acetone for 1–2 seconds. Acetone–alcohol mixture for 10 seconds can also be used for declourization
- Wash slide with tap water
- Counter stain smear with basic fuchsin for 30 seconds. Dilute carbol fuchsin can also be used instead of basic fuchsin
- Wash with tap water

- Wipe carefully around the section to remove as much water as possible, dehydrate quickly in absolute alcohol, clear in xylol or benzol and mount in Canada balsam or DPX.

Mechanism of Gram Reaction

Various theories have been proposed to explain why some bacteria retain the primary stain and some do not.

i. *Cell Wall Permeability Theory*

- According to this theory, the cell wall of Gram-positive bacteria contain more mucopeptide because of which it is thicker and stronger and is impermeable as compared to Gram-negative bacteria.
- During staining with primary stain and mordant dye–iodine complex is formed within cell. Under the action of decolorizing agent, this complex diffuses freely out of the Gram-negative cell but not from the Gram-positive cell because the Gram-positive cell wall is less permeable due to thickness of its cell wall.
- In Gram-negative bacteria mucopeptide is less and therefore their cell wall is relatively less strong and thin, hence dye–iodine complex diffuses out of cell freely and they take up the colour of the counter stain (Saton, 1963).

ii. *Magnesium Ribonucleate Theory*

- According to this theory, presence of magnesium ribonucleate is responsible for Gram-positiveness and its absence is responsible for Gram-negativeness.
- According to this theory, there is a formation of insoluble complex of magnesium ribonucleate—primary stain–iodine complex in Gram-positive bacteria, which is not soluble in decolourizer and it is not removed by alcohol or acetone.
- Thus, Gram-positive bacteria retain the primary stain. As magnesium ribonucleate is absent in Gram-negative bacteria, there is a formation of complex containing primary stain and iodine only, which is soluble in decolourizer and is removed by alcohol or acetone from Gram-negative bacteria and hence are unable to retain primary stain.

iii. *Lipid Content Theory (Stern Theory)*

- This is a more recent theory.
- According to this theory Gram-positive bacteria contain only 4% lipids in their cell walls whereas Gram-negative bacteria contain 20% lipids.
- The high percentage of lipids in Gram-negative bacteria is responsible for Gram-negativeness.
- When primary stain and mordant are applied to smear, both Gram-positive and Gram-negative bacteria are stained violet in colour.
- This is due to formation of dye–iodine complex in both Gram-positive and negative bacteria.
- Subsequently, when the smear is treated with alcohol or acetone for decolourization, the lipid present in the cell wall of Gram-negative bacteria is removed from cell wall because of its solubility in alcohol or acetone.
- This leads to formation of numerous and large size pores in Gram-negative bacteria that results in removal of dye-iodine complex formed in Gram-negative cells.
- Thus, Gram-negative bacteria loose the primary stain and they become colourless and take the counter stain applied later.
- However, in Gram-positive bacteria when decolourizer is applied, the result is dehydration of Gram-positive cells because of fewer lipids and decrease in the pore size of cell wall.
- This results in the reduction of permeability of the cell wall and the dye–iodine complex gets trapped within the Gram-positive cells because of fewer lipids and, they thus retain the violet colour.

iv. *Acid Protoplasm Theory*

- According to this theory, Gram-positive bacteria retain the primary stain more strongly than Gram-negative bacteria.
- Gram-positive bacteria have more acidic cytoplasm than Gram-negative bacteria. Thus, have more affinity towards the basic dyes (primary stains used in Gram staining). Also

the iodine makes the cytoplasm more acidic and acts as a mordant, increasing the attraction of the primary stain to the cell cytoplasm.
- It thus helps to fix the stain in bacterial cell which is why Gram-positive bacteria are able to retain primary stain.
- As the cytoplasm in Gram-negative bacteria is basic in nature; hence, there is no attraction between basic cytoplasm and basic stain; and hence, are unable to retain primary stain.

v. *Isoelectric Point Theory*

- Isoelectric point is the pH where ionization of amphoteric compound is at maximum.
- Isoelectric point range of Gram-positive organisms is pH 2–3, while that of Gram-negative organisms is pH 4–5.
- There are more unsaturated acids in Gram-positive organisms than Gram-negative organisms.
- These unsaturated acids are oxidized during iodine treatment and more acidity (lowered isoelectric point) is produced in the cytoplasm.
- Thus, Gram-positive organisms are able to retain basic dyes at a higher hydrogen ion concentration.

Limitations (Factors Affecting) of Gram Staining

- The Gram reaction is not hard and fast distinguishing feature. It may vary with the age of culture, pH of the medium, viability of the microbes, and choice of the stains. The Gram-positive microbes may appear Gram-negative and Gram-negative microbes may appear Gram-positive.
- The gram reaction depends on the age of the cell. Old cultures of Gram-positive bacteria may readily get decolourized and appear Gram-negative. Old culture of more than 24 hours may contain large number of dead, dying and degenerative cells in which the physical and chemical properties are altered (where cell walls may be weakened). Gram-negative cells are usually observed in a smear of Gram-positive microbes, the number increases with the age of culture. This is particularly true when these microbes are cultivated in media containing fermentable substances that become acidic

in reaction as growth proceeds. It is a characteristic feature of some bacteria, which tend to appear Gram-negative when grown in acidic medium.

- Damage to cell wall due to antibiotic therapy or excessive heat fixation of the smear makes them to appear Gram-negative. Gram-positive cells affected by cell wall active agents such as lysozyme or antibiotics may become Gram-negative. Gram-positive bacteria such *Actinomyces, Arthobacter, Corynebacterium, Mycobacterium,* and *Propioni-bacterium* have cell walls particularly sensitive to breakage during cell division, resulting in Gram-negative staining of these cells. In cultures of *Bacillus* and *Clostridium,* a decrease in peptidoglycan thickness during cell growth may cause some of them to appear Gram-negative.

- Certain group of bacteria can display variable response to the stain, which can be due to growth stress (e.g. unsuitable nutrients, temperatures, pH, or electrolytes) that results in a number of nonviable cells making some bacteria Gram-negative in a Gram-positive culture, but certain bacterial species are known for their Gram variability even under optimal growth conditions.

- Loss of cell walls in Gram-positive bacteria may render them Gram-negative (L-forms). Bacteria totally devoid of cell wall (*Mycoplasma*) are always Gram-negative. Bacteria such as *Mycobacterium* that have extra waxy content in their cell wall are difficult to stain. Small and slender bacteria such as *Treponema, Chlamydia, Rickettsia* are often difficult to stain by Gram's method. Gram-positive bacteria that have been phagocytosed by polymorphs may also appear Gram-negative.

- Some Gram-positive bacteria may lose the stain easily and therefore appear as a mixture of Gram-positive and Gram-negative bacteria (gram-variable). When over-decolourized, even Gram-positive bacteria may appear pink and when under-decolourized Gram-negative bacteria may appear Gram-positive.

- Death of bacteria makes Gram-positive bacteria to appear Gram-negative. Dead Gram-positive bacteria are often stained as Gram-negative.

- Other reasons include:
  - Use of iodine solution which is very old, i.e. yellow in colour instead of brown may affect the gram reaction, which is not able to act as an effective mordant.
  - When a smear is too thick, Gram-negative organisms may not be completely decolourized because of overcrowding of cells and may appear Gram-positive.

Modifications of Gram Stain (Table 6.1)

The original method of Gram's is modified by different workers. The different modifications of original method of Gram are:

Table 6.1: Modifications of Gram stain	
Name of modification	*Particulars of modification*
1. Burke's modification	Decolourization with acetone or acetone– ether mixture
2. Kopeloff and Bermann's modification	Methyl violet as primary stain, acetone as a decolourizer and basic fuchsin as counter stain
3. Jensen's modification	Methyl violet as primary stain and neutral red as counter stain
	Sandiford's counter stain (malachite green) for *Neisseria* species
4. Weigert's modification	Carbol gentian violet—primary stain aniline xylol—decolourizer
	Carmalum—counter stain
5. Preston and Morrell's modification	Ammonium oxalate—crystal violet— primary stain, Lugol's iodine—mordant, Iodine—acetone as decolourizer
	Dilute carbol fuchsin—counter stain
6. Hucker's modification	Aqueous methyl violet or crystal violet— primary stain, acetone—decolourizer, aqueous neutral red/safranin–counter stain
7. Brown and Brenn modification	Aqueous crystal violet or methyl violet– primary stain, acetone and 95% ethanol– decolourizer, 0.5% aqueous safranine/ dilute carbol fuchsin—counter stain.

1. Burke's Modification

Burke in 1922 modified the original method of Gram by using the acetone (100%) or acetone–ether mixture as decolourizer instead of absolute alcohol.

2. Kopeloff and Bermann's Modification (1922)

- This is a modification of Burke's method. In this modification, the staining solutions used were methyl violet with sodium bicarbonate in distilled water as a primary stain, iodine dissolved in 4% NaOH solution as a mordant, instead of alcohol, acetone (100%) as a decolourizer and basic fuchsin as counter stain.
- This method is sometimes modified by substituting acetone–alcohol in the place of pure acetone as a decolourizer. A mixture of acetone and alcohol is recommended because it decolourizes more rapidly than 95% ethanol alone and is less likely to cause over decolourization smears than acetone without the addition of alcohol. This method is recommended for general use.

3. Jensen' Modification

- Jensen used methyl violet as primary stain, iodine and potassium iodide in water as mordant, absolute alcohol as decolourizer and neutral red as counter stain.
- Safranine or basic fuchsin can also be used as a counter stain instead of neutral red, but not the carbol fuchsin as it stains Gram-negative microbes so intensely that they may appear Gram-positive.
- Neutral red is recommended for *Neisseria* spp. because it stains well the *Neisseria* spp. This method is recommended for routine bacteriological work and has been used in examination of exudates for gonococci and meningococci.
- This method, especially when used for gonococci and meningococci, is further modified by using Sandiford's counter stain containing malachite green (malachite green 0.05 gm, pyronine 0.15 gm added to 100 ml of distilled water), particularly when organisms are scanty.

4. Weigert's Modification

- This modification is particularly useful for staining tissue sections and may be used to stain *Pneumocystis* cysts.
- This modification uses carbol gentian violet prepared using saturated alcoholic solution of gentian violet and 5% phenol solution as a primary stain.
- Gram's iodine is used as a mordant and aniline-xylol is used as a decolourizer.
- The counter stain carmalum (carminic acid and potassium alum in water), is used before the application of primary stain.

5. Preston and Morrell's Modification (1962)

- The primary stain used in this modification is ammonium oxalate–crystal violet.
- The smear is washed in Lugol's iodine and further treated with iodine solution.
- The smear is decolorized using iodine–acetone decolourizer and counterstained using dilute carbol fuchsin solution.
- Dilute carbol fuchsin (1 in 10) is recommended for staining of Vincent's bacteria, Yersinia, Haemophilus, Campylobacter, Vibrio spp., etc.

6. Modified Preston and Morrell's Method

- A disadvantage of Preston and Morrell's method is that an irritant aerosol is produced when the iodine–acetone is expelled onto the slide through a jet of a 'squeeze' bottle.
- The acetone quickly evaporates from the droplets and leave minute, airborne nuclei of iodine which when numerous are highly irritating to the eyes and nose. Hence, this method can be further modified to overcome the irritating iodine in aerosols by reducing the iodine concentration to one-tenth and shortening the duration of decolourization to ten seconds.

7. Brown and Brenn Modification

- This modification is used for staining of *Nocardia* and *Actinomyces* species in tissues, and also for staining of fungi.

- This method uses 0.5% aqueous crystal violet or methyl violet solution as primary stain, equal parts of acetone and 95% ethanol as decolourizer and 0.5% aqueous safranine or dilute carbol fuchsin as a counter stain.

8. *Other Modifications*

- **Hucker's modification:** In this method, 1% aqueous methyl violet or crystal violet is used as primary stain, Gram's iodine as a mordant, acetone as a decolourizer and 2% aqueous solution of neutral red or safranin as a counter stain.
- **Gram staining for the colour-blind:** Instead of safranin, pyronin or fuchsin, smear is counterstained with Bismarck brown for 30–60 seconds. Gram-positive organisms are stained purple in colour and Gram-negative organisms are stained yellowish brown in colour.

Applications of Gram Staining

- It differentiates bacteria into Gram-positive and Gram-negative. This differentiation is the first step towards classification of bacteria.
- It is also the first step towards identification of bacteria in cultures.
- Observation of bacteria in clinical specimens provides a vital clue in the diagnosis of infectious diseases.
- Useful in estimation of total count of bacteria.
- Empirical choice of antibiotics can be made on the basis of Gram's stain report.
- Choice of culture media for inoculation can be made empirically based on Gram's stain report.

Miscellanea

- Although Gram stain is useful in staining bacteria, certain fungi such as *Candida and Cryptococcus* are observed as Gram-positive yeasts.
- Half-Gram stain refers to modified staining technique, where the smear is neither decolorized nor counterstained. It is useful to stain a known Gram-positive bacterium.

- Rapid Gram stain refers to quick technique where the smear is exposed only for 30 seconds instead of one minute.
- In specimen such as sputum, capsulated bacteria may stand out as clear spaces between the bacterium and the pink (mucus) background.
- The spores may stand out as clear, unstained region in spore forming bacteria.
- The acid-fast bacteria, *Mycobacterium tuberculosis* in particular is difficult to stain by Gram stain and is considered as an example of gram neutral, although it is weakly Gram-positive in nature.

7 Differential Staining II: Ziehl-Neelsen Staining
(Acid-fast Staining)

- The microorganisms such as *Mycobacterium tuberculosis, Mycobacterium leprae,* atypical mycobacteria and others, which do not get stained easily with ordinary staining method but once stained they resist decolourizing action of dilute mineral acids are called acid-fast microorganisms and method used for staining of these microorganisms is known as acid-fast stain.

- It is a differential staining method, which differentiates acid-fast organisms (mycobacteria) from others (non-acid-fast).

- Acid fastness is due to the high content of lipids, fatty acids and higher alcohols, which constitute almost 40% of the dry weight of acid-fast microorganisms.

- The cell wall of certain bacteria and parasites is able to bind with fuchsin dye because of high lipid content (mycolic acid—a long chain fatty acid containing 50–90 carbon atoms) and hence, they are not destained by acid–alcohol as mycolic acid helps them to resist decolourization by acid and alcohol and makes them acid as well as alcohol fast.

- The ordinary aniline dye solutions do not readily penetrate the substance of the acid-fast microorganisms and are therefore unsuitable for staining of acid-fast micro-organisms. However, by using powerful staining solution containing phenol and application of heat, the primary stain can be made to penetrate and stain the acid-fast microorganisms.

HISTORY

- **Koch** in 1882 stained *Mycobacterium tuberculosis* with hot alkaline methylene blue as the primary stain and vesuvin as the decolourizer and counter stain.
- **Paul Ehrlich** (1882) discovered the acid-fast property. He used hot fuchsin in the presence of aniline oil as a mordant and destaining with a dilute nitric acid.
- **Ziehl** changed the mordant to phenol and **Neelsen** combined the mordant with primary stain to form carbol fuchsin.
- These modifications suggested by **Ziehl-Neelsen** (1882, 1883) were described by **Johne** (1885), hence it is known as Ziehl-Neelsen staining method.
- **Kinyouns** in 1915 developed a cold staining method for acid fast bacilli. Various alternate methods have been devised by different workers, e.g. Cooper modification, Gabbett modification and Muller-Chermock carbol fuchsin—Tergitol cold stain method.

STAINING REAGENTS

Ziehl-Neelsen (Strong) Carbol Fuchsin (Primary Stain)

Basic fuchsin	10 gm
Absolute alcohol (ethanol 95%)	100 ml
5% phenol (5 gm phenol in 100 ml distilled water)	1000 ml

- Dissolve basic fuchsin in ethanol. Mix 100 ml of alcoholic basic fuchsin and 1000 ml 5% phenol solution.
- Alternatively dissolve the basic fuchsin in the phenol by placing them in a flask over a boiling water-bath for about 5 minutes, shake the contents from time to time.
- When solution is complete, add alcohol to it and mix thoroughly. Then add distilled water to it and mix.
- Filter the mixture before use.

Kinyoun's Carbol Fuchsin

Basic fuchsin	4 gm
95% ethanol	20 ml

Distilled water	100 ml
Phenol crystals	8 gm

- Dissolve basic fuchsin in ethanol.
- Add distilled water slowly while stirring.
- Melt phenol crystals with gentle heat and add to basic fuchsin solution.

20% Sulphuric Acid (Decolourizer)

- Concentrated H_2SO_4 (250 ml) and distilled water (1000 ml).
- Take Distilled water in a flask and add concentrated H_2SO_4 slowly over 10 minutes down the side of flask into the cold water.
- Never add water to acid.
- *Alternatives*
  a. 3% HCl acid in 95% alcohol (industrial methylated spirit).
  b. Concentrated HCl (3 ml) and 95% alcohol (97 ml).
  c. 25% H_2SO_4 for 2–4 minutes—used in revised national tuberculosis control programme (RNTCP).
  d. 20% H_2SO_4 for one minute followed by 70% alcohol for 2–3 minutes.

95% Alcohol (Secondary Decolourizer)

Ethanol (95 ml) and water (5 ml).

Methylene Blue (Counter Stain)

- Loeffler's methylene blue is used.
- It is prepared by adding saturated solution of methylene blue in alcohol (300 ml) and 0.01% KOH in water (1000 ml).
- **Alternatives for methylene blue**
  a. *Malachite green* is the best among the counter stains used. It gives a pale green colour to background—useful if the observer is colour blind and also it is pleasant for eyes. Use 1% aqueous solution of malachite green.
  b. *Picric acid* gives yellow colour to background useful if the observer is colour-blind and a counter-stain for exceptionally thick smears as it does not stain background so intensely. It also has advantage of not selectively

staining the cellular material. Dissolve 0.75 gm of picric acid to 100 ml of fresh distilled water or use a saturated solution of picric acid.

c. **Brilliant green:** Gives green colour to the background. Dissolve 0.01 gm of NaOH in 100 ml of distilled water, dissolve 1 gm brilliant green. If colour is intense at this concentration then dilute this 1:20 with distilled water or use 0.5% aqueous solution of brilliant green.

Procedure

- Prepare smear on a clean glass slide, allow it to air dry and fix it by flaming.
- *Alcohol fixation of smear:* Fixation of smear by using alcohol is recommended when the smear is not prepared from sodium hypochlorite (bleach) treated sputum and will not be stained immediately. *M. tuberculosis* is killed by bleach and during the staining process. Heat fixation of untreated sputum is not recommended as it does not kill *M. tuberculosis* in smear. Alcohol fixation is recommended as it is bactericidal in nature and able to kill *M. tuberculosis* in smear.

Primary Staining

- Cover the whole slide and not only the smear with carbol fuchsin filtered through Whatman filter paper no. 1 and heat gently from below until steam rises.
- The whole slide is covered with stain to avoid uneven heating and cracking of the slide while heating.
- Avoid boiling of primary stain; allow it to act for 5–10 minutes with intermittent heating.
- The stain should never be allowed to boil otherwise stain deposits will be formed which may give erroneous results.
- The stain must not be allowed to evaporate and dry on the slide.
- If necessary, add more stain to the slide to cover the smear and reheat. Heating is necessary for penetration of stain into the cell wall.
- Heat and phenol from carbol fuchsin help the primary stain to penetrate through the cell wall.

- Wash the slide with tap water.
- Alternatively, exposure of smears to carbol fuchsin for 15–60 minutes at temperature ranging from 37° to 80°C has also been reported.

Decolourization

- Cover the slide with 20% sulphuric acid (H_2SO_4).
- The red colour of the smear changes to yellowish brown.
- After about 1 minute wash the slide with water and observe the colour of the smear, if it is red, repeat decolourization till it becomes very faintly pink or yellowish brown.
- The process of decolorization may take a total time of 10 minutes. Then wash with water.
- Revised National Tuberculosis Control Programme (RNTCP) advocates use of 25% H_2SO_4 as a decolourizer for *M. tuberculosis*. Use of 25% H_2SO_4 for 2–4 minutes as a decolourizer and washing with water is recommended. If smear is not properly decolourized by this, 25% H_2SO_4 is applied again for 1–3 minutes to ensure complete decolourization.
- The smear can be treated with secondary decolourizer, i.e. 95% ethanol for 2 minutes.
- This step is optional and can be omitted, if specimen is not urine.
- The basis of this practice is the fact that tubercle bacilli are alcohol-fast as well as acid-fast. Advantages of this step are:
  - Decolourization is completed more quickly and the margins and underside of the slide are more completely cleaned and freed from deposits of the stain.
  - It decolourizes certain atypical acid fast bacteria, e.g. *M. smegmatis*, a harmless commensal in the regions of urethral orifice from urine samples is only acid-fast but not alcohol fast, may be encountered in pathological specimens and otherwise be confused with tubercle bacilli, are decolorized with 95% ethanol. *M. smegmatis* may cause confusion in the diagnosis of renal tuberculosis, if secondary decolourization is not carried out.
- Wash with water.

Counter Staining

- Counter stain with methylene blue or malachite green for 1–2 minutes.
- Wash, blot dry with clean paper and air dry the slide before observing under oil immersion objective.
- Observe under 100X after putting a drop of cedarwood oil.

Observations

- Acid-fast bacilli appear bright red, straight or slightly curved rods, occur singly or in small groups, may appear beaded rods (beaded forms are seen as they are stained unevenly whereas atypical mycobacteria are stained evenly) (Fig. 7.1).
- Pus cells, epithelial cells and other microorganisms appear blue or green.

REPORTING

- At least 10,000 acid-fast bacilli should be present per ml of the sputum for them to be demonstrable in direct smears.
- A negative report should not be given till at least 300 fields have been examined, taking about 10 minutes.

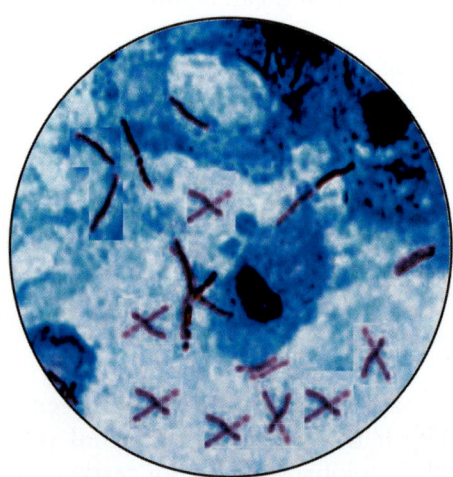

Fig. 7.1: Acid-fast bacilli

- A positive report can be given only if 2 or more typical bacilli have been seen.
- When no AFB are seen after examining 300 fields—the smear is to be reported as **no AFB seen.** It should not be reported as **negative** as organisms may be present in the smear but might have not been seen in those fields, which have been examined.
- Two specimens—one collected preferably as an early morning specimen should be examined.

Grading of smear		
No. of AFB	*Seen in (oil immersion field)*	*Report*
0	300	AFB not seen
1–2	300	doubtful, repeat smear
1–9	100	1+
1–9	10	2+
1–9	1	3+
10 or more	1	4+

STAINING OF TISSUE SECTION

Procedure

- Treat the tissue section mounted on the slide with xylene to remove paraffin.
- Wash well with alcohol and then with water.
- Apply carbol fuchsin and allow it to act as in routine procedure but heat the slide gently to avoid detachment of section from the slide.
- Apply 20% H_2SO_4 as in routine procedure for decolourization.
- Decolourize smear with alcohol.
- The process of decolourization takes longer time because of the thickness of the section.
- Wash smear carefully to avoid dislodgement of the section.
- Counter stain with methylene blue or malachite green for 30–60 seconds.
- Wash with water.

- Blot dry the slide and section carefully.
- Flush the slide with absolute alcohol, wipe the slide again and clear in xylene.
- Mount in Canada balsam or DPX.
- Observe under the oil immersion objective.

Examples of AFB (Microbes Stained by ZN Staining)

Bacteria

- Mycobacteria—*Mycobacterium tuberculosis, M. leprae,* atypical mycobacteria.
- Species of *Nocardia* and *Rhodococcus* are partially acid-fast.
- *Legionella micdadei*—causative agent of pneumonia is partially acid-fast in tissues.
- *Yersinia pseudotuberculosis.*

Parasites

- *Cryptosporidium, Cyclospora* and *Isospora* are distinctly acid-fast
- *Taenia saginata* egg

Microbial Structures

- Bacterial spores
- Fungal spores

Modifications of ZN Staining

Any modification in the acid-fast staining where different percentages of H_2SO_4 (other than 20% H_2SO_4) is used is known as modified acid-fast staining.

a. Leprosy bacilli are also acid-fast but are weakly acid-fast and can be decolourized with 5% H_2SO_4.

b. 10% H_2SO_4—for *Cryptosporidium* spp.

c. 1% H_2SO_4—for *Nocardia* spp., *Actinomycetes*

d. 1% H_2SO_4 is used as decolourizer to demonstrate acid-fastness of tissue sections containing clubs formed by Actinomycetes, Nocardia and mycobacteria.

e. 0.25–0.5% H_2SO_4—for bacterial spores.

f. 25% H_2SO_4—for *M. tuberculosis* under RNTCP.

g. Kinyoun's cold method—for *Cryptosporidium* spp.

h. Muller-Chermock carbol fuchsin—Tergitol cold stain.

i. Cooper modification.

j. Gabbett modification.

Hot and Cold Staining Techniques

- In the hot staining technique, the phenolic solution of basic fuchsin stain is heated to enable the stain to penetrate the waxy coat of mycobacterial cell wall.

- In the cold staining technique, the primary stain is not heated. In cold staining technique, penetration of the primary stain is usually achieved by increasing the concentration of basic fuchsin and phenol, and incorporating a **wetting agent** chemical.

Kinyoun's Cold Stain Method (for *Cryptosporidium* spp.)

i. Cover smear with Kinyoun's carbol fuchsin stain. Keep it for 5 minutes without heating. Rinse slide with distilled water.

ii. Decolorize with acid-alcohol (3 ml of HCl + 97 ml of 95% alcohol) for 3 minutes. Rinse with distilled water.

iii. Repeat decolourization until no red color appears in the wash. Rinse with distilled water.

iv. Counter stain with methylene blue for 1 minute. Rinse slide with distilled water. Air dry. Do not blot.

Kinyoun's Stain Method for Nocardia Species and Fungal Elements

- Prepare smear on a clean glass slide and fix the smear by gentle heating.

- Flood the smear with Kinyoun's carbol fuchsin solution.

- Allow the slide to stand for 20 minutes.

- Wash the smear with tap water.

- Decolorize the smear with 1% sulfuric acid until no more colour appears in the washing (approximately 1 minute).

- Rinse with tap water.

- Counter stain with methylene blue for approximately 1 minute.
- Rinse with tap water and air dry.

Observations

- The filaments of *Nocardia* species and *Rhodococcus* appear red-stained against a blue background.
- The hat-shaped ascospores of *Pichia anomala* appear pink in colour.

Cooper Modification

- Cover fixed smear with Cooper's carbol fuchsin (100 ml carbol fuchsin used in ZN stain + 3 ml of 10% NaCl solution—keep in refrigerator) for 3–5 minutes with gentle heating
- Wash with distilled water
- Decolourize smear with 5% nitric acid in 95% alcohol
- Wash with distilled water
- Counter stain with Cooper's brilliant green for 30 seconds or longer
- Wash with distilled water
- Dry and examine

Gabbett Modification

- Stain smear with carbol fuchsin
- Wash with distilled water
- Decolourize and counter stain smear at a same time for 2 minutes with Gabbett methylene blue containing 2 gm of methylene blue and 100 ml of H_2SO_4—filtered after 24 hours (or 1 gm of methylene blue + 20 ml of H_2SO_4 + 30 ml of absolute alcohol + 50 ml of distilled water).
- Wash with distilled water
- Dry and examine

Mueller-Chermock Carbol Fuchsin— Tergitol Cold Stain Method

- Cover fixed smear with carbol fuchsin containing one drop Tergitol no. 7 (sodium heptadecyl sulfate) to each 25 ml stain.

- Allow it to act for 2 minutes without heating.
- Wash with tap water.
- Decolourize smear with acid–alcohol until the smear becomes colourless.
- Wash with water.
- Counter stain with methylene blue approximately for 5–15 seconds depending on thickness of smear.
- Wash with water.
- Dry and observe.

Hot Modified Acid-fast Stain for *Cryptosporidium* in Stool

- Cover heat fixed stool smear with carbol fuchsin.
- Heat to steaming and allow to act stain for 5 minutes.
- Rinse with water.
- Decolourize smear with 5% aqueous H_2SO_4 for 30 seconds.
- Rinse smear with water.
- Counter stain with methylene blue for 1 minute.
- Wash with water.
- Dry and observe.

Brucella Differential Stain

- It is used to demonstrate *Brucella abortus* in infected tissues or exudates (placental material and other products of abortion).
- This method may also be used to demonstrate *Coxiella burnetii* and Chlamydiae in tissue sections.
- In this method, 1:10 diluted carbol fuchsin is allowed to act without heating for 15 minutes and then decolourized with 0.5% acetic acid for 15 seconds.
- Washed thoroughly with water.
- Counter stained with Loeffler's methylene blue for 1 minute.
- Observe under oil immersion objective.

Observations

- *Brucella abortus* appears red or orange in colour.
- Other pathogens—*Coxiella burnetii* and Chlamydiae in tissue sections also show similar appearance.

Mechanism of Acid-fast Stain

- Acid-fast organisms are not easily stained because they are coated with lipids, fatty acids and higher alcohols in their cell wall.
- Mycolic acids (waxy substance)—long chain, multiple cross-linked fatty acids present in the cell wall do not allow the stain to penetrate easily inside these organisms.
- In ZN staining carbol fuchsin (basic fuchsin, phenol)—a phenolic solution of basic fuchsin is applied with heat. Heat and phenol facilitate penetration of the dye.
- Subsequently, when decolourized by acid, the dye does not come out because it is soluble in phenol and phenol is more soluble in lipid substances (mycolic acid); hence, there is no decolourization and they retain the colour of the basic fuchsin (primary stain).
- The process of decolourization removes the primary stain (carbol fuchsin) from the background cells, tissue fibres and other organisms in the smear except for acid-fast organisms.

Important Points

Staining of AFB may be facilitated and stain can be made to penetrate in several ways as follows:
- By using powerful staining solution containing phenol.
- By application of heat.
- By increasing the concentration of phenol and basic fuchsin in primary stain.
- By prolonged contact of primary stain and smear.
- By adding wetting agent such as Tergitol.

Important Precautions

1. To minimize cross-contamination of smears on slides
   - Fix smears properly
   - Stain slides individually or on rack where they may be kept separated
   - Wipe oil immersion lens with lens paper after examining each slide

2. To prevent contamination of slides or stains with extraneous environmental AFB
   - Prepare all staining reagents with fresh distilled water
   - Check tap water, distilled water reservoirs and delivery tips for AFB
   - Do not use reagents that are too old
   - Use positive and negative control smears as a check on reagents and staining.

Important Observations

- Number of AFB required in per ml of sputum to give positive results.

  It has been estimated that when using standard concentration technique, approximately 10,000 AFB/ml are required to detect microscopically or to give positive results by direct microscopy.

- Staining properties of virulent strains of *Mycobacterium tuberculosis.*

  Virulent strains of MTB are strongly acid-fast in nature than avirulent strains of MTB. The virulent strains can be distinguished from non-virulent on the basis of amount of stain taken up by the cells.

8

Differential Staining III: Romanowsky Stains

- Romanowsky staining is a permanent staining method commonly used for demonstration of haemoparasites—parasites found in the blood smears (blood parasites).
- This staining method is developed by Romanowsky in 1891 for staining of malarial parasites.
- The original Romanowsky stain was prepared by dissolving the compound formed by the interaction of watery solutions of eosin and zinc-free methylene blue in methyl alcohol.
- This original stain is replaced by various modifications, which are easy to use and also they give better results than original method.
- The different modifications include:
  1. Leishman's stain
  2. Wright's stain
  3. Giemsa stain
  4. Field's stain
  5. Jenner's stain
  6. Jaswant Singh-Bhattacharya (JSB) stain
- These stains are of two types:
  i. Type one stains include Leishman and Wright stains which contain both fixatives and staining reagents. Hence, fixation of thin smear and tissue smear is not required. However, thick blood smears need to be dehaemo-globinized.
  ii. Type two stains include Giemsa, Field and JSB stains which contain staining reagents only and no fixative is present. When any of these staining methods is used, the tissue smear and thin blood smears/films are need to be fixed before staining by using methanol.

- The typical property of the Romanowsky stains is that they impart a reddish-purple colour to the chromatin of malarial and other parasites stained by these methods.
- This typical reddish-purple colour is due to a substance, which forms when methylene blue is ripened.
- For ripening—two methods are used:
  i. *Slow ripening method by age:* The stain is ripened slowly for 12 months or more. The stain is kept in bottles, which are half-filled and shaken at intervals to aerate thoroughly the contents. This method is used for polychrome methylene blue.
  ii. *Quick ripening method:* The stain is ripened quickly by heating with sodium carbonate. This method is used in Leishman's and Wright's stains.
- The ripened methylene blue is mixed with an aqueous solution of eosin.
- The resultant precipitate formed due to the combination of these two stains is washed with distilled water, dried and dissolved in pure methyl alcohol.
- This combination of methylene blue and eosin also contains oxidation products of methylene blue called azures, which provide further contrast in peripheral blood smears.
- Each modification of the Romanowsky stain varies according to the ripening and the relative properties of methylene blue and eosin.
- Romanowsky stains are water-based and methanol-based stains.
  - In methanol-based stains, e.g. Leishman's stain, the stock solution prepared in pure methanol is not diluted before use.
  - In water-based stains, e.g. Giemsa, Field's and JSB, the stock solution is diluted with distilled water (pH 7.0–7.2).

LEISHMAN'S STAIN

Staining Reagent

Leishman's powder—150 mg
Methanol (pure)—100 ml

- Dissolve the Leishman's powder in a dark bottle.
- Shake well until the powder is dissolved completely.
- The stain matures in next two days; hence, allow stain to stand for 48 hours with intermittent shaking.
- Alternatively the readymade staining solution (ready to use) commercially available may be purchased and used.

Procedure

- Staining of thin blood smears/films
  - Prepare thin blood smear on a clean glass slide.
  - Cover the smear with 5 to 10 drops of the stain and allow it to act for 2 minutes.
  - Add 10 to 20 drops of buffered distilled water (pH 7.2), i.e. double the quantity of stain and mix by gently rocking the slide.
  - Allow the diluted stain to act for 10 to 15 minutes.
  - Wash with buffered distilled water until the smear appears bright red in colour.
  - Dry the slide by placing it upright.
  - First screen the smear under the low-power objective (10X) of the microscope for detection of microfilaria and observe at least two hundred microscopic fields using 100X objectives for the presence of malarial parasites.
- Staining of thick blood smears/films
  - The thick blood smear is dehaemoglobinised by immersing the slide in water until red colour disappears.
  - After the process of dehaemoglobinisation is completed, the smear is stained—steps of staining are same as that for staining a thin smear.
  - After staining, air dry the film in a vertical position.
  - Observe the stained smear under oil immersion objective (100X) for detection of malarial parasites and microfilaria.
- Staining of tissue sections
  - To remove the paraffin, treat the section with xylene, then with ethyl alcohol and finally with distilled water.

- Drain off the excess water and cover section with a mixture of 1 part Leishman's stain and 2 parts distilled water or buffer solution and allow it to act for 5–10 minutes.
- Wash with distilled water.
- Differentiate with a weak solution of acetic acid (1 in 1500), controlling the differentiation under the low power of the microscope until the protoplasm of the cells is pink and only the nuclei are blue.
- Wash with distilled water or buffer solution.
- Blot, dehydrate with a few drops of absolute alcohol, clear in xylene and mount in Canada balsam or preferably DPX mounting medium.

Observations (Fig. 8.1)

- Cytoplasm of WBCs and protozoal parasites appear blue in colour
- Nuclei, parabasal body and flagella of protozoal parasites appear red in colour
- Nuclei and granules of PMNs appear purple in colour
- RBCs appear pink in colour
- Granules of eosinophils appear pink in colour

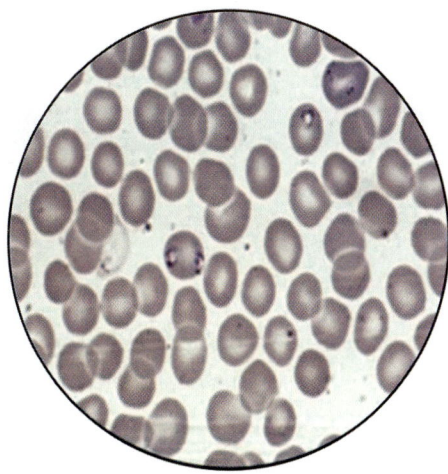

Fig. 8.1: Leishman's stained smear showing malarial parasites

WRIGHT STAIN

Staining Reagent

Wright stain powder	0.3 gm
Glycerol	3 ml
Absolute methyl alcohol	7 ml

- Mix Wright stain powder with 3 ml of glycerol with the help of a mortar and pestle.
- Mix this solution, after being grinded well, with 7 ml of absolute methyl alcohol.
- Store this mixture/staining solution in amber glass-stoppered bottle.
- Always filter this solution before use.

Procedure

- Cover the blood smear with 5–10 drops of Wright's stain and allow it to act for 1 minute.
- Add 10–20 drops of buffered distilled solution and mix well with the staining solution.
- Rinse slide with buffered distilled water, dry and observe under the microscope.

Observations

Same as in Leishman's stain.

GIEMSA'S STAIN

Staining Reagent

Giemsa stain powder	0.75 g
Glycerol	25 ml
Methanol (pure)	75 ml

- Place Giemsa stain powder in a mortar.
- Add glycerol and grind with a pestle until a paste is formed.
- Add methanol and mix well.
- Heat this staining solution in a dark-colored bottle in an incubator at 37°C for 24 hours.

Procedure

i. *Rapid Method*

The rapid method is used for staining blood smears for demonstration of blood parasites.

For thin blood smears

- The blood smear is fixed with absolute methyl alcohol for 2–3 minutes or absolute ethanol for 15 minutes.
- Allow blood smear to dry.
- The smear is stained with a mixture containing 1 part of Giemsa's stain and 10 parts of buffered distilled water (pH 7.2) and allow it to act for 30–60 minutes.
- Wash with buffer solution.
- Allow the slide to drain by keeping it in upright position and dry the slide in air.
- Observe under the oil immersion lens (100X).

For thick blood smear

- Do not fix the smear with methanol.
- Rest of the staining steps are same as that for staining a thin smear.
- Observe under the oil immersion lens.

Observations (Fig. 8.2)

Same as in Leishman's stain

Advantages

- This method gives excellent results with thin blood smears for malarial parasites—Schuffner's dots are well defined by using this stain.
- This method is also very good for demonstration of trypanosomes.

ii. *A Modified Rapid Method*

- A rapid method with the application of heat for fixation of smear instead of methyl alcohol may be used for demonstration of Spirochaetes.
- In this method, the smear is fixed by drawing slide three times through a flame.

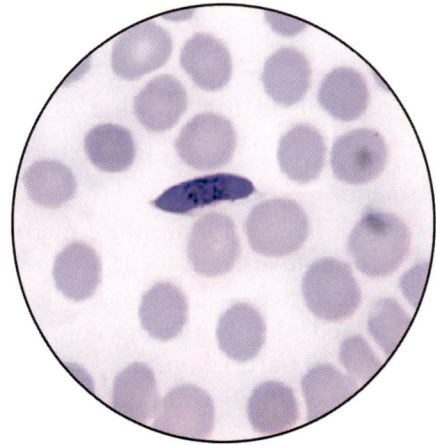

Fig. 8.2: Giemsa's stained smear showing malarial parasites

- Alternatively, smear can be fixed by applying absolute alcohol for 15 minutes.
- Prepare a fresh solution 10 drops Giemsa's stain solution with 10 ml of buffer solution-(pH 7.0) and mix well by shaking.
- Apply this staining solution to fixed smear.
- Warm till steam rises, allow to cool for 15 seconds and then pour off.
- Apply fresh stain and heat again.
- Repeat the procedure for 4–5 times.
- Wash in distilled water, allow to dry and mount.
- Observe under oil immersion lens (100X).

iii. *Slow Method*

- The slow method is used for demonstration of microbial objects which are difficult to stain by rapid methods, e.g. some pathogenic Spirochaetes.
- The principal is to allow the diluted stain to act for a longer period.

Procedure

- Fix the smear in methyl alcohol for 3 minutes.
- In a Petri plate, mix 1 ml of Giemsa stain with 20 ml of buffer solution (pH 7.0).

- Place a piece of thin glass rod in the stain in the Petri plate.
- Place the smear in a Petri plate with one end resting on the glass rod with the smear side downwards.
- Ensure that there is sufficient stain between the smear and the bottom of the Petri plate.
- In this way, allow stain to act for 16–24 hours.
- Wash the slide in a stream of buffer solution.
- Allow smear to dry in air, mount and observe under oil immersion lens (100X).

JENNER'S STAIN

Staining Reagent

Jenner's stain powder   5 gm
Methanol   1000 ml

- The Jenner's stain is a mixture of several thiazin dyes.
- The Jenner's stain powder is taken into a conical flask to which methanol is added.
- The mixture is warmed to 50°C.
- It is to be mixed properly by shaking several times during the day.
- After 24 hours, it is to be filtered and used.
- No ripening is required.

Procedure

- Prepare smear on a clean glass slide and allow it to dry.
- Apply absolute methanol for 15–30 seconds and then drain.
- Apply one ml of Jenner's stain and allow it to act for 3 minutes.
- Add one ml of phosphate buffer solution (pH 6.6) and one ml of deionized water to smear, and allow it to stand for 45 seconds.
- Rinse smear with deionized water.
- Allow it to dry in air.
- Observe under the microscope.

JSB (JASWANT SINGH-BHATTACHARYA) STAIN

This method uses two staining reagents.

Staining Reagents

JSB 'A' (eosin)

Eosin	2.5 gm
Distilled water	100 ml

JSB 'B' (methylene blue—azure)

Methylene blue—azure	2.5 gm
Distilled water	100 ml

Procedure

1. *For thin blood smears*
   - Fix the blood smear by immersing the slide in methanol for 2 minutes.
   - Allow the slide to dry in air by placing it upright.
   - Immerse the slide in JSB 'A' solution (5 ml of JSB 'A' stock solution and 70 ml of distilled water filtered) for 5 minutes.
   - Allow it to drain thoroughly in a vertical position and allow it to air dry.
   - Immerse the slide in JSB 'B' solution for 30–60 seconds.
   - Wash the slide by dipping it in water (pH 6.2 to 6.6) for 2–4 seconds.
   - Allow it to drain thoroughly in a vertical position and allow it to air dry.
   - Observe under the oil immersion lens (100X).

2. *For thick blood smear*
   - The steps of staining thick smears are same as for thin films except that the smear is not fixed with methanol.
   - The omission of this step allows lysis of RBCs and dehaemoglobinisation by the aqueous staining solution.
   - After the staining procedure is completed dry the slide by placing it upright.
   - Observe under oil immersion lens (100X).

FIELD'S STAIN

Staining Reagents

- *Solution 'A' (methylene blue—azure)*

Methylene blue	0.4 g
Azure 1	0.25 g
Buffered water (solution 'B')	250 ml

- *Solution 'B' (buffered water)*

$Na_2HPO_4.12H_2O$	25.2 g
KH_2PO_4	12.5 g
Distilled water	1000 ml

- *Solution 'C' (eosin)*

Eosin	0.5 g
Buffered water (solution 'B')	250 ml

Procedure

1. *For thin smear*
   - Fix the smear by immersing the slide in methanol for 2 minutes.
   - Allow slide to dry by placing it upright.
   - Dip the slide in solution 'A' for 1–3 seconds.
   - Rinse the slide in solution 'B' for 2–3 seconds.
     - Dip the slide in solution 'C' for 1–3 seconds.
     - Dry the slide by placing it upright.
2. *For thick smear*
   - Slide is not fixed with methanol.
   - Other steps are same as that for staining of a thin smear.
   - Observe smear under the oil immersion lens (100X).

9

Impregnation Staining

INTRODUCTION

- Organisms like Spirochaetes and fine structures of bacteria like flagella are difficult to see under light microscope as they are beyond the resolving power of the light microscope.
- These structures which are too thin to be seen under ordinary microscope, can be rendered visible by increasing their thickness by impregnating silver on their surface.
- Impregnation of silver on slender objects artificially thickens them with a deposit of silver (silver-plated) and make them appear larger than the actual.
- The silver solution used in the impregnation technique is not a stain. It is a metallic salt that differs from stain in following respects:
  - It is a colourless
  - It is stable and do not fade
  - It is opaque
  - It precipitates on the surface of object
  - It is not observed like stain
  - It is deposited on the surface of object and thereby increases its thickness
  - Its deposit is densely black and hence, gives good contrast.

SILVER SOLUTIONS

- Ammoniated silver solutions are used as they are easily reduced.
- Different silver solutions can be used. Silver nitrate is the most commonly used silver salt. Other silver salts, which can be used include: Silver diamine, silver carbonate, etc.

Uses

- This method is used for demonstration of Spirochaetes and bacterial flagella.
- Fontana's method, Levaditi's method and Faulkener and Lillie's method are the examples.
- Fontana's staining method is the most commonly used impregnation staining method for the staining of Spirochaetes, especially the smaller Spirochaetes like treponemes and leptospires.

1. FONTANA'S METHOD

Staining Reagents

i. *Fixative*

Acetic acid	1 ml
Formalin (40%)	2 ml
Distilled water	100 ml

Mix them together

ii. *Mordant*

Phenol	1 gm
Tannic acid	5 gm
Distilled water	100 ml

Mix phenol crystals and tannic acid in distilled water.

iii. *Ammoniated Silver Nitrate*

- Add 10% ammonia to 0.5% solution of silver nitrate in distilled water.
- Go on adding it until the precipitate formed just dissolves.
- After the precipitate dissolves, add more silver nitrate solution drop by drop till the precipitate reappears and does not re-dissolve.

Staining Procedure

- It is used for staining of films.

- The steps in staining procedures are:
  - Preparation of a film on glass slide.
  - Treatment of film with the fixative for three times, 30 seconds each time.
  - Washing of slide with absolute alcohol and it is allowed to act for 3 min.
  - Drain off the excess alcohol and carefully burn off the remaining alcohol until the film becomes dry.
  - Treat with mordant, heat the film till the steam rises and allow it to act for 30 seconds.
  - Wash with distilled water and again dry the film/slide.
  - Treat the film with ammoniated silver nitrate, heat the film till the steam rises and allow it to act for 30 seconds.
  - When the film becomes brown in colour, wash well in distilled water, dry it and mount in Canada balsam under a cover-slip, as some immersion oils may cause the film to fade at once.
  - Allow it to air dry and observe under microscope (100X).

Observations

- Spirochaetes appear brownish-black (Fig. 9.1)
- Background—brownish-yellow.

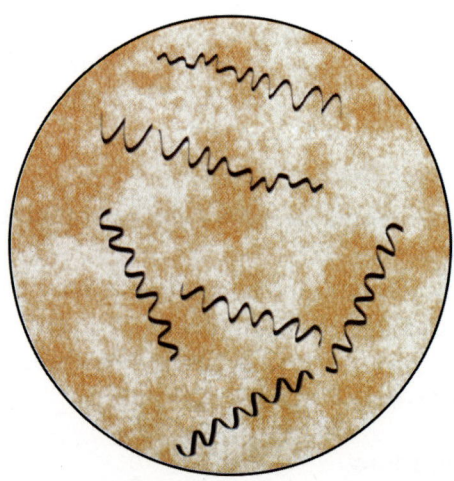

Fig. 9.1: Fontana's stain showing Spirochaetes

Mechanism

The deposition/impregnation of silver salt on the surface of Spirochaetes increases their thickness with the help of mordant, which helps in binding of silver salt to the Spirochaetes.

2. LEVADITI'S METHOD

- It is used for staining of Spirochaetes in tissues.
- This method is a modification of original Fontana's method.
- It uses pyridine.
- It is more rapid method than the original one.

Procedure

- Small pieces of tissue, around 1 mm thick, are fixed in 10% formalin for 24 hours.
- Wash the tissue with water for 1 hour.
- Washed tissue is placed in 96–98% alcohol for 24 hours.
- Tissue is placed in a 1% silver nitrate solution containing one-tenth of the volume of pure pyridine for 2 hours at room temperature and later on at about 50°C for 4–6 hours.
- The tissue is rapidly washed with 10% pyridine solution.
- The tissue is placed in reducing fluid (containing 100 parts of 4% formalin to which pure acetone—10 parts and pure pyridine—15 parts, are added immediately before use) and kept in this fluid for 2 days at room temperature in the dark.
- The tissue is washed well with water and then dehydrated with increasing strengths of alcohol.
- The fixed tissue is embedded in paraffin wax.
- Thin sections, around 5 μm thick, are cut with the help of a microtome.
- The sections are mounted on slide.
- The slide is treated with xylene to remove paraffin.
- After removing the paraffin, the sections are immediately mounted on Canada balsam.

10

Staining of Spores

- Spore is highly resistant resting phase of bacteria, which is impermeable to ordinary stains.
- When spore forming organisms are stained by ordinary staining methods or Gram staining method, the bacterial body is coloured deeply but spore is not stained.
- It remains unstained and appears as a clear area.
- To visualize spore more clearly, it is necessary to introduce staining reagent into the substance of the spore.
- Hence, spores are stained using special staining methods.
- Special staining is a staining method used to stain (to colour) specific parts of bacterial cells, e.g. staining of endospores, capsule, cell wall, granules, etc.
- Different special staining methods are used to stain the spores. These include:
  - Modified Ziehl-Neelsen staining method
  - Schaeffer and Fulton's staining method
  - Dorner's method
  - Wirtz-Conklin method
  - Abbott method

1. MODIFIED ZIEHL-NEELSEN STAINING METHOD

A modified ZN staining method using 0.25% or 0.5% sulphuric acid, instead of 20% used for staining of *M. tuberculosis*, can be used for staining of bacterial spores.

Procedure

- Prepare a thin film on glass slide, dry it in air and fix it by minimum amount of dry heat.

- Apply Ziehl-Neelsen's carbol fuchsin for 3–5 minutes with application of heat from below until steam rises.
- Wash in water.
- Treat smear with 0.25% or 0.5% sulphuric acid for one to several minutes.
- Wash with water.
- Alternatively, smear can be decolourized with 2% nitric acid in absolute ethyl alcohol. For decolourization the slide is dipped once rapidly in this solution and immediately washed in water. This gives better results.
- Counter stain smear with 1% aqueous methylene blue for 3 minutes.
- Wash with water, blot dry and observe under 100X.

Observations

- Spores appear bright red in colour
- Bacterial body appears blue in colour (Fig. 10.1)

Special Note

Lipid granules, if present in the cytoplasm, may stain dark red in colour and may appear like small spherical spores.

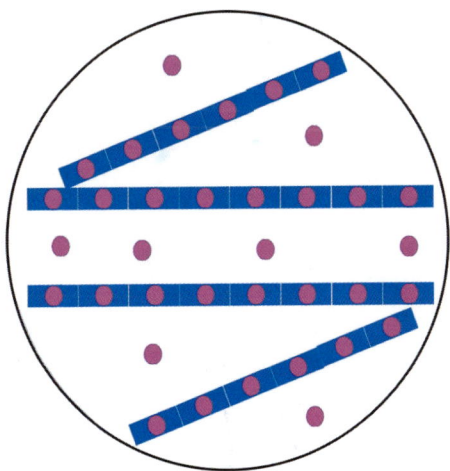

Fig. 10.1: Bright red-coloured spores stained by modified ZN staining

Examples of Sporulating Bacteria

- *Bacillus* spp.—aerobic bacilli
- *Clostridium* spp.—anaerobic bacilli
- *Sporolactobacillus* spp.—anaerobic bacilli
- *Sporosarcina* spp.—cocci

2. SCHAEFFER AND FULTON'S STAINING METHOD

This method was developed by Schaeffer and Fulton, and modified by Ashby in 1938.

Procedure

- Prepare smear on clean glass slide, allow it to air dry and fix it by minimal flaming.
- Place the slide over a beaker of boiling water, resting it on the rim.
- When large condensed droplets appear on the underside of the slide, flood the smear with 5% aqueous solution of malachite green and allow it to act for 1 minute, or
- Alternatively, flood the smear with hot malachite green and allow it to act for 1 minute.
- Wash with cold water.
- Counter stain with 0.5% safranine or 0.05% basic fuchsin for 30 seconds.
- Wash, dry and observe under 100X.

Observations

- Spores appear green in colour
- Bacterial body appears—red in colour (Fig. 10.2).

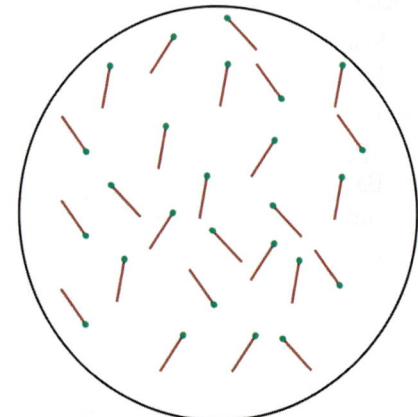

Fig. 10.2: Green-coloured spores stained by Schaeffer and Fulton's staining method

Special Note

Lipid granules are not stained by this method and appear colourless.

3. DORNER'S METHOD

This method uses Kinyoun carbol fuchsin used in cold staining method.

Procedure

- Make a heavy suspension of organisms in 3–4 drops of distilled water in a test tube.
- Add equal volume of freshly filtered Kinyoun carbol fuchsin.
- Place test tube in boiling water bath for 5–10 minutes.
- Take a drop of 10% aqueous solution of nigrosin on a glass slide.
- Take a loopful of suspension of organisms from tube and mix with nigrosin.
- Prepare a thin smear by spreading.
- Dry the smear quickly by gentle heating and observe under 100X.

Observations

- Spores appear pink in colour
- Bacterial body appears colourless
- Background appears dark gray in colour (Fig. 10.3).

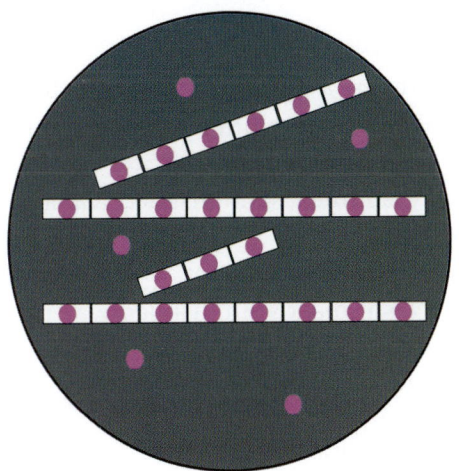

Fig. 10.3: Pink-coloured spores stained by Dorner's method

4. MODIFIED DORNER'S METHOD

In this method, the procedure of staining is modified.

Procedure

- Prepare smear on glass slide and fix it.
- Cover smear with a strip of filter paper.
- Apply carbol fuchsin-steam for 5–7 minutes.
- Remove filter paper.
- Wash with water and blot dry.
- Cover smear with a thin film of nigrosin using another slide or a needle.

Observations

- Spores appear pink in colour
- Bacterial body appears colourless
- Background appears dark gray in colour.

5. WIRTZ AND CONKLIN METHOD

It is another staining method used for staining of spores.

Procedure

- Prepare a thin smear on glass slide and fix it by flaming.
- Flood smear with 5% aqueous malachite green and steam 3–6 minutes.
- Wash smear with distilled water.
- Apply 0.5% aqueous safranine or 0.5% merbromin (mercurochrome) for 30–60 seconds.
- Wash smear with distilled water.
- Allow it to dry.
- Observe under 100X.

Observations

- Spores appear green in colour
- Bacterial body appears pink in colour.

6. ABBOTT STAIN

This is another method used for staining of spores (Fig. 10.4).

Procedure

- Prepare a thin smear on glass slide and fix it by flaming.
- Apply saturated alcoholic solution of methylene blue (prepared by rubbing up of 1.5 gm of methylene blue with 100 ml of 95% alcohol in mortar), or
- Apply Manson methylene blue (2 gm of methylene blue ground in borax solution containing 5 gm of sodium tetraborate crystals in 100 ml of distilled water).
- Apply heat from below till the methylene blue stain boils.
- Repeat heating for several times but not continuously for one minute.
- Wash smear with distilled water.
- Cover smear with a mixture of one part of saturated alcoholic eosin Y solution and nine parts of distilled water for 5–10 seconds.
- Rinse smear with distilled water.
- Blot and dry the smear.
- Mount it in balsam and observe under the microscope.

Observations

- Spores appear blue in colour (Fig. 10.4).
- Bacterial body appears pink in colour.

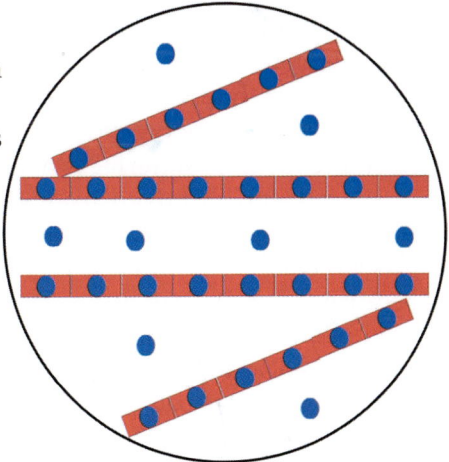

Fig. 10.4: Blue-coloured spores stained by Abbott stain

11

Staining of Capsule

INTRODUCTION

- Bacterial capsule is a loose, gelatinous, amorphous layer around the cell wall.
- When loosely and irregularly arranged, it is called slime layer and when organized into sharply defined structure, it is known as capsule.
- When the capsule has a width of more than 0.2 (20 nm) and can be seen under the light microscope, it is called macro-capsule.
- When the capsule has a width of less than 0.2 (20 nm) and cannot be seen under light microscope, it is called microcapsule.

PRINCIPLE

- Capsule contains 98–99% of water and 1–2% of solids—generally a polysaccharide, but in some bacteria it may be a glycoprotein or a polypeptide.
- As the capsular material is water-soluble and may be displaced and removed by vigorous washing, capsule staining is very difficult as compared to other special staining procedures.
- Because of non-ionic nature of capsule, the stains commonly used are unable to bind with capsule. Hence, two staining reagents—acidic and basic are used to stain. The acidic stain is used to stain the background and the basic stain is used to stain the bacterial body.
- Bacterial capsules appear as unstained halos surrounding the bacterial bodies, when stained by ordinary staining

methods. Hence, special staining methods are used for their demonstration.
- Two types of staining methods are used to demonstrate capsule. These include:
  - Negative staining methods
  - Positive staining methods

Negative Staining Methods

- In this staining, the background is stained and the capsule is seen as unstained hollow surrounding the bacterial body.
- Two types of negative staining methods can be used. These are:
  1. The wet film India Ink method
  2. Dry film negative staining method.

1. The Wet Film India Ink Method

- This is the best method for staining of capsules on bacteria in the liquid as well as solid media.
- In this, the capsule displaces the colloidal carbon particles of the India ink and appears as a clear hallow around the bacterial body.

Procedure

- Take a clean glass slide free from particles of dust or girt.
- Place a large loopful of undiluted India ink on the glass slide.
- Take a small portion of solid bacterial culture or a small loopful of liquid bacterial culture in the India ink and emulsify.
- In case of solid culture, need to rub the speck of solid material on the surface of glass slide just beside the drop of the India ink before mixing it into the India ink.
- Take a clean grit-free cover slip and place on the ink drop and press it down so that the film becomes very thin and appear pale in colour.
- Observe immediately under 40X as well as 100X by reducing the intensity of light. The intensity of light can be reduced by lowering the condenser considerably.

Observations

- Background—black/dark
- The capsule—clear refractile halo around the bacterium
- The capsule is seen as a clear space between the highly refractile outline of the bacterium and the dark/black background of ink particles.

Advantages

i. This is the most simple method and readily practicable; hence, most suitable.
ii. As the smear is not dried and fixed, there is no shrinkage of capsule; hence, it is clearly apparent even when narrow.
iii. It is the best method for demonstration of capsule on bacteria from liquid as well as solid media.

Disadvantage

This is not a permanent preparation; hence, cannot be fixed and stored for longer duration.

Special Precaution

The India ink should be dense, homogenous, very finely granular and should not be contaminated with capsulated or non-capsulated bacteria.

2. Dry Film Negative Staining Method

- This method uses India ink, nigrosin or eosin.
- It is a permanent preparation that can be fixed and stored for longer duration.

Procedure

- Place a loopful of 6% of glucose in water at one end of a slide.
- Add small amount of bacterial culture to this and mix it properly.
- Add a loopful of India ink, nigrosin or eosin to the drop and mix it.
- Spread the mixture over the slide in the form of a thin film with the help of another slide.
- Allows it to air dry.

- Fix smear by using Leishman stain or methyl alcohol.
- Do not fix smear by heating. Heating of smear causes cell shrinkage that may create a clear zone around the bacterium—an artifact that may be mistaken for capsule.
- Drop on Gram's methyl violet and allow it to act for 1–2 minutes.
- Wash in water.
- Blot and dry.
- Observe smear under 100X.

Observations (Fig. 11.1)

- Bacterial body—dark violet
- Capsule seen as a clear zone between bacterium and the dark ink background.

Advantage

It is a permanent preparation. Hence, can be fixed and stored for longer duration.

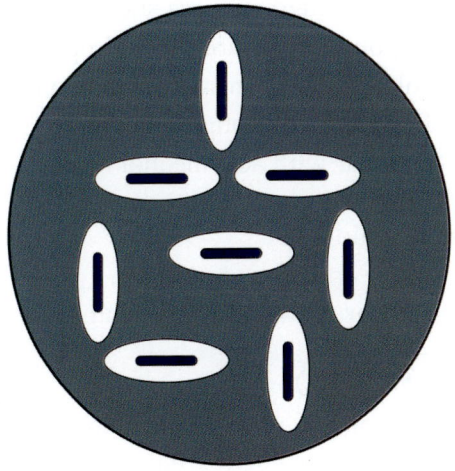

Fig. 11.1: Bacterial capsule—dry film negative staining method

Disadvantages

i. This is a less reliable method, as the shrinkage spaces give the appearance of capsules around non-capsulated bacteria.

ii. Occasionally, capsules may be shrunken or obscured and may be rendered invisible.

Congo Red Capsule Stain

- It is a modification of the nigrosin negative stain.
- The bacteria are stained pink with Congo red and the background is stained then with acid fuchsin.
- The capsule or slime layers do not stain—exclude both stains.
- The bacterial cells are stained pink, and the capsules appear as clear halos.

Staining Reagents

- Congo red
- Acid fuchsin
- Alcohol

Procedure

- Place a loopful of Congo red on a slide.
- Mix a small amount of culture to the drop of Congo red.
- Spread the culture and stain suspension on the slide.
- Allow the slide to dry thoroughly in air.
- Fix the dried smear with acid alcohol for 15 seconds.
- Rinse with distilled water and cover the slide with acid fuchsin for 1–5 minutes.
- Rinse with water and allow to air dry.
- Observe the smear under oil immersion lens (100X).

Observations (Fig. 11.2)

- Bacterial body appears red/pink in colour
- Capsules appear as colorless halos against a dark blue background.

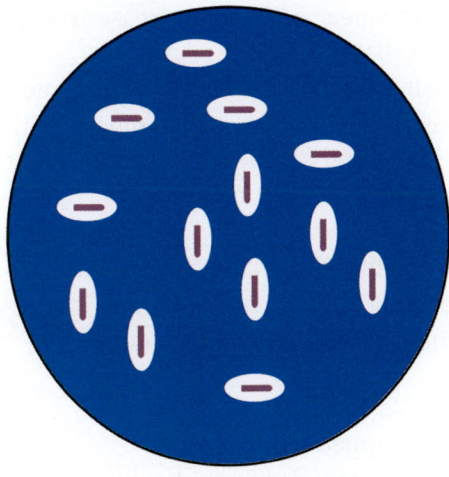

Fig. 11.2: Bacterial capsule—Congo red capsule stain

Positive Staining Methods

- In these methods, the capsule is stained and coloured.
- The positive staining methods are less reliable and hence, are generally not recommended.
- These staining methods include:
  1. Hiss method
  2. MacNeal method
  3. Lawson method
  4. Anthony method
  5. Muir's method
  6. Howie and Kirkpatric method

1. Hiss Method

Staining Reagents

- *Hiss stain:* Mix 5 ml of saturated alcoholic solution of gentian violet in 95 ml of distilled water. Alternatively, 1% crystal violet can be used.
- 20% copper sulphate solution.

Procedure

- Mix bacterial suspension with a drop of normal serum and then use for smear preparation.

- Prepare a thin smear on a clean grease-free glass slide and allow it to air dry.
- Fix smear using alcohol or 1:10 diluted commercial formalin.
- Cover smear with Hiss stain or 1% aqueous solution of crystal violet and heat gently it from below until steam just begins to rise.
- Allow stain to act for 1 minute.
- Wash off the stain with a 20% copper sulphate solution.
- Wipe the back of slide, clean and allow it to dry in air.
- Observe under oil immersion lens (100X).

Observations

- Bacterial body appears dark purple
- Back ground appears dark purple
- Capsule appears pale blue or pale lavender in colour

2. MacNeal Method

Staining Reagents

MacNeal Tetrachrome stain

Eosin Y	1 gm
Methylene blue	1 gm
Azur A	0.6 gm
Methylene violet	0.2 gm
Acetone-free neutral methyl alcohol	1000 ml

- Mix well the ingredients and heat to 50°C for 30 minutes.
- Keep at 37°C for 2 days with intermittent shaking for several times.
- Filter through filter paper.

Procedure

- Prepare a thin smear on a clean glass slide.
- Allow smear to dry in air.
- Cover smear with MacNeal tetrachrome stain for 3–5 minutes.
- Wash carefully with distilled water.
- Dry it in air and observe under oil immersion lens (100X).

Observations
Capsule appears colourless or pale in colour.

3. Lawson Method
Staining reagents

i. *Lawson mordant*
It is a 5% solution of phosphomolybdic acid prepared using distilled water.

ii. *Lawson stain*
Wright stain   10 ml
Glycerin   5 ml
Glycerin is to be added to Wright stain just prior to use.

Procedure
- Prepare a direct smear from the culture on a clean glass slide without using a diluent.
- Allow it to dry in air.
- Cover smear with Lawson mordant and allow it to act for 30 seconds.
- Wash smear with methyl alcohol.
- Cover smear with 20 drops of Lawson stain and allow it to act for 2 minutes.
- Add 30 drops of distilled water, mix stain on slide with water and allow to act for 10–20 minutes.
- Rinse with distilled water.
- Drain slide, allow to air dry and observe under oil immersion lens (100X).

Observation
Capsules appear colourless or pale.

4. Anthony Method

Staining Reagents
i. Aqueous crystal violet solution—1%
ii. Copper sulphate solution—20%

Procedure

- Prepare a thin and even smear with skimmed milk or litmus milk by spreading with the help of another glass slide.
- Allow it to air dry and fix it by heating.
- Apply 1% aqueous crystal violet solution and allow it to act for 2 minutes.
- Wash smear with 20% copper sulphate solution.
- Allow it to air dry and observe under oil immersion lens (100X).

Observations

- Background appears purple
- Capsules appear unstained against purple background.

5. Muir's Method

Staining Reagents

  i. *Solution I (primary stain)*
     Ziehl-Neelsen's carbol fuchsin
 ii. *Solution II—Muir mordant*

20% aqueous solution of tannic acid	2 parts
Saturated aqueous solution of mercuric chloride	2 parts
Saturated aqueous solution of potassium alum	5 parts

iii. *Solution III* (counter stain)
     Methylene blue   0.3%

Procedure

- Prepare a thin smear on a clean glass slide.
- Allow it to dry in air.
- Cover smear with a piece of filter paper of size of smear.
- Apply solution I and heat slide from below with Bunsen flame until steam rises for 30 seconds.
- Rinse gently with 95% ethanol and then with water.
- Apply solution II (Muir mordant) and allow it to act for 15–30 seconds.
- Wash well with water.
- Decolourize smear with ethanol for 30 seconds or till the smear becomes faint pink in colour.

- Apply solution III (counter stain) for 30 seconds.
- Wash with water.
- Allow it to air dry and observe under oil immersion lens (100X).

Observations
- Bacterial body appears red in colour
- Capsules appear blue in colour

6. Howie and Kirkpatric Method

Staining Reagents

10% water-soluble eosin or erythrocin in distilled water	4 parts
Human, rabbit, sheep or ox serum (heated to 56° for 30 minutes) + crystals of thymol	1 part

- Store the mixture at room temperature for several days, centrifuge and retain the supernatant fluid stain.
- Store it at room temperature for several months.

Procedure
- Take a drop of culture suspension or pathological exudates with the help of inoculation loop of diameter of 1 mm on a clean glass slide.
- Mix it with one drop of eosin solution and leave it for about 1 minute.
- Spread this mixture with the help of edge of another slide as in the preparation of blood smear.
- Allow it to air dry.
- Observe under the oil immersion objective (100X).

Observations
- Bacterial body appears red in colour.
- Capsules appear lightly stained or remain unstained.
- Background appears red in colour.

12

Staining of Granules

INTRODUCTION

- Inclusion granules are non-living bodies deposited in the cell cytoplasm.
- These are not permanent and essential structures and are present in some species of bacteria.
- These are sources of stored energy.
- These may be present as lipid, polysaccharides (starch or glycogen), polymetaphosphate (volutin) and sulphur granules.

STAINING OF VOLUTIN GRANULES

- Volutin granules are also called metachromatic granules because they exhibit the phenomenon of metachromasia in which a stain of a particular colour stains a cell component with different colour than its original colour. This colour shift is called metachromasia.
- This property is very commonly exhibited by volutin granules and hence, are named as metachromatic granules.
- Volutin granules are polymetaphosphate in nature and are also known as **Babes Ernst granules**, polar bodies and metachromatic granules.
- These are present in *Corynebacterium diphtheriae* (diphtheria bacillus), other species of *Corynebacterium* and some species of *Bacillus*.
- These granules can be seen in unstained wet preparations as round refractile bodies in the cytoplasm.

- When stained with basic dyes, they stain more strongly than the rest of the bacterial body.
- They show the phenomenon of metachromasia, i.e. when they are stained with toluidine blue or methylene blue, they appear reddish purple in colour.
- They are more clearly demonstrated by special staining methods such as:
  1. Albert's stain
  2. Neisser's stain
  3. Ljubinsky's stain
  4. Gohar's stain
  5. Methylene blue stain
  6. Ponder's stain

1. ALBERT'S STAIN

- Devised by Albert; hence, named as Albert's stain.
- This original method devised by Albert is modified by Laybourn in 1924 in which methyl green (originally used by Albert) is substituted with malachite green.
- This method is named as **Albert-Laybourn method** and is recommended for routine use.

Principle

The volutin granules exhibit a property of metachromasia, i.e. they appear in a colour which is different from the original colour of the stain. Hence, when they are stained with toluidine blue present in staining solution of Albert's stain, they appear bluish-black in colour.

Staining Reagents

Staining Solution (Albert's Stain I)

Toluidine blue	1.5 gm
Malachite green	2 gm
Glacial acetic acid	10 ml
Alcohol (95% ethanol)	20 ml
Distilled water	1000 ml

- Dissolve toluidine blue and malachite green in the ethanol, add to the water and acetic acid.
- Allow the mixture to stand for one day and then filter.

Albert's Iodine (Albert's Stain II)

Iodine	6 gm
Potassium iodide	9 gm
Distilled water	900 ml

- Potassium iodide is added to 10 ml of water and then iodine is added.
- Finally, the distilled water is added.

Procedure

- Prepare a smear on clean glass slide either from exudates collected from pseudomembrane or from colony of *C. diphtheriae* grown on culture media.
- Allow smear to dry in air and then fix by passing slide 2–3 times gently over the flame.
- Cover the smear with Albert's stain I and allow it to act for 3–5 min.
- Wash smear in water and blot dry.
- Cover the smear with Albert's stain II and allow it to act for 2–3 min.
- Wash with water and blot dry.
- Observe it under the oil immersion lens (100X).

Observations (Fig. 12.1)

- Granules appear bluish-black in colour
- Bacterial body appears green in colour
- Other organisms appear light green in colour

2. NEISSER'S STAIN

Procedure

- Prepare smear on a clean glass slide, allow it to air dry and fix it by heat.
- Stain with Neisser's solution for 30–60 seconds.
- Wash with distilled water.

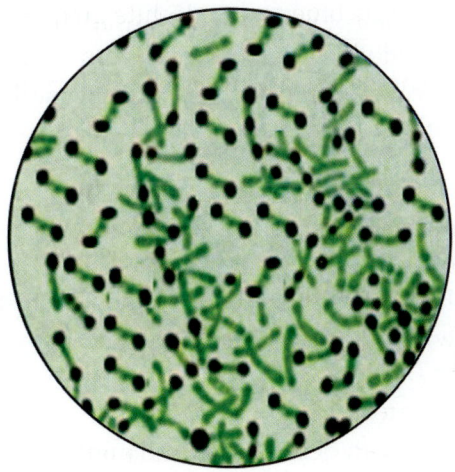

Fig. 12.1: *Corynebacterium diphtheriae* showing metachromatic granules (Albert's stain)

- Apply Bismarck brown for 10 seconds.
- Wash with distilled water.
- Dry in air and observe under oil immersion lens (100X).

Observations
- Metachromatic granules appear black in colour
- Bacterial body appears light green in colour

Neisser's Stain (Modified)
Staining reagents
    i. *Neisser's methylene blue*

Methylene blue	1 gm
Ethyl alcohol	50 ml
Glacial acetic acid	50 ml
Distilled water	1000 ml

- Dissolve methylene blue in alcohol in a mortar.
- Mix acetic acid with distilled water and then add to methylene blue solution slowly.
- Filter after 24 hrs.

ii. *Iodine solution:* One which is used in Kopeloff and Beerman's modification of Gram stain

iii. *Neutral red solution:* One which is used in Jensen's modification of Gram stain.

Procedure

- Prepare smear on a clean glass slide, allow it to air dry and fix it by heat.
- Apply Neisser's methylene blue and allow it to act for 3 min.
- Wash off with dilute iodine solution and allow it to remain on slide for 1 min.
- Wash with water.
- Counter stain with neutral red for 3 min.
- Wash in water and dry.
- Observe under oil immersion lens (100X).

Observations (Fig. 12.2)

- Granules appear deep blue in colour
- Bacterial body appears pink in colour

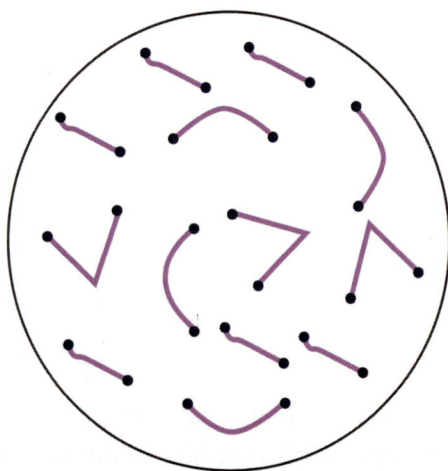

Fig. 12.2: *Corynebacterium diphtheriae* showing metachromatic granules (Neisser's stain)

3. LJUBINSKY STAIN

Staining Reagents

i. Ljubinsky Stain

Crystal violet	0.25 gm
Glacial acetic acid	5 ml
Distilled water	95 ml

ii. Bismarck Brown

Bismarck brown Y	0.2 gm
Distilled water	100 ml

- Dissolve Bismarck brown Y in boiling distilled water and filter while it is still hot.

Procedure

- Apply Ljubinsky stain and allow it to act for 3 min.
- Wash with distilled water.
- Apply Bismarck brown and allow it to act for 30 seconds.
- Wash with distilled water and dry.
- Observe under oil immersion lens (100X).

Observations

- Granules appear deep purple in colour
- Bacterial body appears brownish in colour

4. GOHAR'S METHOD

Staining Reagents

i. Methylene Blue Stain

Methylene blue	1.5 gm
95% alcohol	100 ml

- Grind methylene blue in small amount of alcohol in a mortar.
- Mix this with alcohol.
- Store in glass-stoppered bottle.
- Filter after 24 hrs.

Procedure

- Apply methylene blue and allow it to act for 5 min.
- Quickly decolourize smear with 1:1000 sulfuric acid.
- Rapidly wash with water.
- Apply Gram's iodine for 10 seconds.
- Counter stain with 1% eosin in distilled water for 30 seconds.
- Wash with distilled water.
- Dry in air and observe under oil immersion lens (100X).

Observations

- Granules appear dark in colour.
- Bacterial body appears yellowish in colour.

5. METHYLENE BLUE STAIN

Staining Reagents

Methylene blue stain

Methylene blue	0.3 gm
10% potassium hydroxide	0.1 ml
95% alcohol	30 ml
Distilled water	100 ml

- Grind methylene blue with alcohol in a mortar, then transfer to flask.
- Wash mortar with a mixture of potassium hydroxide added to distilled water.
- Add washings to flask.
- Filter after 24 hrs.

Procedure

- Apply methylene blue to smear for 1–2 min.
- Wash with distilled water.
- Dry in air and observe under oil immersion lens (100X).

Observations

- Metachromatic granules appear deep blue in colour.
- Bacterial body appears light blue in colour.

6. PONDER'S METHOD

It is a staining method described by Ponder for staining of diphtheria bacilli using a weak solution of toluidine blue.

Procedure

• It is a hanging drop preparation in which smear is prepared on a clean cover-slip to which a loopful of the stain is applied.
• Then a cover-slip is inverted over a slide and observed as a hanging drop.

Observations

• The granules are stained sharply and appear dark ruby red in colour.
• Other bacilli are stained faintly.

Modified Ponder's Stain

Staining Reagents

Toluidine blue	0.1 gm
Azure 1	0.01 gm
Methylene blue	0.01 gm
Acetic acid (glacial)	1 ml
Alcohol (95%)	5 ml
Water	120 ml

Procedure

• Prepare smear from specimen or culture on a clean glass slide in the usual manner.
• Fix smear with heat by passing through the flame in the usual manner.
• Cover smear with stain and allow it to act for two minutes or more.
• Wash with water.
• Allow it to dry.
• Observe under oil immersion lens (100X).

Observations

- The granules appear clear and sharp, and are stained dark red in colour.
- Bacterial body is stained pale blue in colour.
- Other bacilli are stained pale.

STAINING OF LIPID GRANULES

1. Burdon's Method (1946)

Staining Reagents

Sudan black stain

Sudan black B powder	0.3 gm
Ethyl alcohol (70%)	100 ml

- Mix, shake thoroughly at intervals and stand overnight before use.

Procedure

- Prepare smear on a clean glass slide, allow it to dry in air and then fix it by heat.
- Cover the smear with Sudan black stain and allow it to act for 15 min at room temperature.
- Drain off excess stain, blot the slide gently with filter paper and dry in air.
- Decolourize smear with the help of xylene. Around 10–15 seconds are required to complete the process of decolourization.
- Allow to air dry or blot dry.
- Counter stain the smear lightly with 0.5% aqueous safranine or dilute carbol fuchsin for 10–15 seconds.
- Rinse with tap water and blot dry.
- Observe under oil immersion lens (100X).

Observations

- Lipid granules appear blue black or blue gray in colour.
- Bacterial body appears pink in colour.

2. Lipid/Spore Stain (Holbrook and Anderson, 1980)

- This is a combined method for staining of lipid granules and bacterial spores.
- It is equivalent to combining Burdon's stain for lipid granules with Ashby's stain for bacterial spores.

Procedure

- Prepare a smear on clean glass slide from the center of a 1-day-old colony or from the edge of a 2-day-old colony.
- Allow it to air dry and fix it with minimal flaming.
- Apply 5% malachite green to smear, place slide on a boiling water in a beaker and allow it to act for 2 min.
- Wash with water and blot dry.
- Apply 0.3% Sudan black B in 70% ethanol for 15 min.
- Wash smear with xylene for 5 seconds and blot dry.
- Counter stain smear with 0.5% safranine for 20 seconds.
- Wash in water, dry and observe under oil immersion lens (100X).

Observations

- Lipid granules appear black in colour
- Bacterial spores appear green in colour
- Cytoplasm appears red in colour.

3. Staining of Polysaccharide Granules/Polysaccharides

- The polysaccharide constituents of bacteria and fungi are stained by periodic acid-Schiff (PAS) method.
- The PAS method can also be used for demonstration of fungal elements in tissue sections.

Periodic Acid–Schiff (PAS) Method

- The polysaccharide constituents of bacteria and fungi are oxidized by periodate to form, which are stained to red-coloured compounds with Schiff's fuchsin-sulphite.
- The proteins and nucleic acids remain uncoloured.

- PAS method also stains fungal elements in infected tissue sections, which are stained as red in colour.
- The tissue material, except glycogen and mucin fails to take the stain.

Staining Reagents

i. Periodic Solution

Periodic acid	1 gm
Distilled water	100 ml

- Dissolve periodic acid in distilled water.
- Use freshly prepared stain.
- If staining solution is protected from light, it can be used for 1–2 days.

ii. Fuchsin–Sulphite Solution

Basic fuchsin	2 gm
Boiling water	400 ml
Hydrochloric acid (2 mol/litre)	10 ml
Potassium metabisulphite	4 gm

- Dissolve basic fuchsin in boiling water, cool to 50°C and filter.
- To the filtrate add HCl and potassium metabisulphite.
- Stopper it and store in a dark cool place overnight.
- Add 1 gm decolourizing charcoal, mix and filter promptly.
- Add up to 10 ml or more HCl until the mixture when drying in a thin film on glass does not become pink.
- Preserve in a stoppered bottle in dark.
- Stain, if stored properly, remains effective for several weeks.

iii. Sulphite Wash

Potassium metabisulphite	2 gm
Concentrated hydrochloric acid	5 ml
Distilled water	500 ml

- It should be freshly prepared reagent.

Procedure

- Prepare smear on a clean glass slide, allow it to air dry and fix it by flaming.

- For tissue sections—fix with usual fixatives, bring to 70% ethyl alcohol and wash thoroughly with this.
- Treat smear/tissue section with periodate solution for 5 min.
- Wash in running tap water for 15 min and rinse in distilled water.
- Apply fuchsin–sulphite and allow it to act for 15 min.
- Wash with sulphite wash solution for two or three times, and rinse in distilled water.
- Apply counter stain—dilute aqueous malachite green or 0.1% light green in 90% alcohol and allow it to act for 1 min.
- For tissue sections—dehydrate rapidly in absolute alcohol, clear in xylene and mount in Canada balsam.

Observations
- Polysaccharide granules appear red in colour
- Polysaccharide constituents of bacteria and fungi appear red in colour
- Fungal elements in tissue sections appear red in colour.

13

Staining of Flagella

INTRODUCTION

- Flagella are very fine structures that cannot be observed under a light microscope as they are beyond the resolving power of ordinary light microscope by using ordinary staining techniques.
- Generally, flagella are demonstrated by electron microscope because of their extreme thinness.
- Metal shadowed films or films made with phosphotungstic acid for negative staining are used for their demonstration under the electron microscope.
- However, when flagella are thickened 10 times by using suitable mordant, they can be made visible under the light microscope by using a special staining techniques.

SPECIAL PRECAUTIONS

- Flagella are very delicate, fragile and heat labile structures; hence, require careful handling during the process of staining.
- For flagella staining, the cultures for smear preparation should be young and vigorous. In general, a 12 to 24 hours growth on surface of agar is satisfactory.
- When stock culture is to be used, make daily subculture for several days.
- Cover slip or slides must be very clean. Special care should be taken to clean. Place in hot cleaning solution, clean in strong sodium or potassium hydroxide, rinse in weak hydrochloric acid and then rinse in distilled water. Keep in

alcohol until ready to use. Burn off alcohol just before use, by holding them in flame with the help of forceps.
- Ensure complete elimination of grease before preparation of smear by placing a tiny drop of culture diluted in distilled water.

PREPARATION OF SMEAR

- Fix the broth culture or saline suspension of colonies from agar plate by adding formalin to give a final formaldehyde concentration of 1–2%.
- Centrifuge at 2000–3000 rpm/min.
- Decant the supernatant liquid and re-suspend the sediment in distilled water by rotating the tube alternately in opposite directions, rolling it between the palms of the hand.
- Centrifuge again and re-suspend in fresh distilled water so as to obtain a final suspension, which is slightly cloudy.
- Take a loopful of material, place it on the clean glass slide and gently spread over an area of 1–2 cm in diameter.
- Allow it to air dry or place the slide in incubator at 37°C.
- Do not fix the smear by heat, it may destroy the flagella.

LEIFSON'S METHOD

Staining Reagents

Leifson stain

Potassium alum in distilled water (5% solution)	10 ml
Tannic acid in distilled water (2% solution)	10 ml
Basic fuchsin in 9% alcohol (1% solution)	10 ml

- Mix them in order.
- Alternatively commercially available flagella stain can be used.
- 1.5 g of commercially prepared stain is dissolved in a mixture of 35 ml of 95% alcohol and 65 ml of distilled water.

Staining Procedure

- With the help of marker pen, mark a heavy line along the edges of the slides, leaving 2 cm on one end free for handling.

- Place a large drop (loopful) of bacterial suspension on one end and tilt the slide so that the bacterial suspension spreads on the slide.
- Allow the smear to dry in air.
- Prepare such three smears on 3 slides.
- Cover smears with 1 ml of Leifson stain and allow the stain to act for 8 min to first smear, 10 min to second smear and 12–15 min to third smear.
- Wash smear with tap water.
- Counter stain with methylene blue (1:1000) in a 1:2000 aqueous solution of borax for 10 min, this step is optional and may be omitted.
- Wash with water, rinse with distilled water, drain and dry in air.
- Observe under oil immersion lens (100X).

Observations

- Flagella appear pink in colour.
- Bacterial body appears blue in colour.

MODIFIED LEIFSON'S STAIN

Staining Reagents

Solution A

Distilled water	100 ml
Sodium chloride	0.75 gm
Tannic acid	1.5 gm

Solution B

Basic fuchsin (special for flagella staining)	0.69 gm or
Pararosaniline acetate	0.45 gm and
Pararosaniline hydrochloride	0.15 gm
Ethyl alcohol (95%)	50 ml

- Shake and keep overnight to dissolve.

Working Solution

- Mix solution A to solution B thoroughly.

- Adjust pH to 5.0 ± 0. 2
- Store in aliquots in suitable container in a frozen state (can be stored for several months).
- For use, take stain from frozen state, allow it to thaw, mix well (as alcohol and water get separated during freezing).
- Store at 4°C (remains stable for 1 month at 4°C).

Procedure

- Inoculate fresh slant culture with motile bacteria, incubate 16–20 hrs at temperature below optimum temperature (generally at room temperature).
- Add 2–3 ml of distilled water by running down the glass side of slant.
- Keep slant at room temperature for 1 hour.
- Transfer 5 or 6 drops of liquid from the butt area with the help of Pasteur pipette to 10% formalin (40% formaldehyde). Make a slightly turbid suspension.
- Take one drop of this suspension on a clean glass slide on one end and incline the slide so that drop slowly spreads on the entire slide.
- Allow smear to dry in air.
- Cover smear with modified Leifson's stain and allow it to act for 10 min.
- Rinse with tap water. Do not pour off stain before rinsing.
- Counter stain with 1% aqueous solution of methylene blue, if needed (this step is optional).
- Wash with water, allow smear to dry in air and observe under oil immersion lens (100X).

Observations

- Flagella appear red in colour
- Bacterial body appears blue in colour

LEIFSON-HUGH MODIFICATION

- Inoculate bacteria to be stained in flagella broth (tryptone, NaCl, dibasic potassium phosphate and distilled water, pH 7.0) in test tubes.

- Incubate it for overnight.
- Add 0.25 ml formaldehyde (40%) to 5 ml of flagella broth culture in a 15 ml centrifuge tube. Mix gently, allow it to stand at room temperature for 15 min.
- Fill centrifuge tube with distilled water, mix well and centrifuge at 2000 rpm for 30 min.
- With the help of Pasteur pipette, remove supernatant carefully without disturbing the pellet.
- Re-suspend pellet gently in 1 ml of distilled water. Again refill the tube with distilled water, mix well and centrifuge at 2000 rpm for 30 min.
- Remove supernatant carefully re-suspend pellet again in 1 ml distilled water.
- Add distilled water slowly until the suspension becomes slightly opalescent.
- Do not invert tube.
- Take a loopful of this suspension on a cleaned glass slide, apply it on slide with appropriate marking.
- Allow smear to air dry. Do not fix it by heat.
- Apply 1 ml of modified Leifson's stain to smear for 5–15 min. After precipitate is observed in staining solution, keep stain on slide for approximately 1 min.
- Wash it on the staining rack till the stain has been completely removed.
- Lift the slide from rack, wipe its back, allow it to dry in air or blot.
- Observe under oil immersion lens (100X).

Observation

Flagella appear red in colour.

SLIVER PLATING STAIN

Staining Reagents

i. *Solution 1—Mordant*

Saturated aqueous solution of aluminium
potassium sulfate   25 ml

| Tannic acid (10%) | 50 ml |
| Ferric chloride (5%) | 5 ml |

- Mix well the above constituents and store the mixture in dark at 5°C.

ii. *Solution 2—Stain*

| Concentrated ammonium hydroxide | 2.4 ml |
| Silver nitrate (5%) | 90 ml |

- Prepare by adding slowly the concentrated ammonium hydroxide to the 5% silver nitrate solution until the brown precipitate re-dissolve.
- Add silver nitrate solution (2–20 ml) dropwise until a faint cloudiness persists.
- Store at 5°C in dark.

Procedure

- Grow bacteria for 16–24 hours at 25°C in motility medium (semisolid agar) or tryptic soy agar (TSA) slant.
- Place 4 loopfuls of sterile distilled water on clean glass slides.
- With the help of inoculating needle (from motility medium) or loop (from the liquid formed at the base of TSA slant) take growth and mix bacteria with distilled water on slides.
- Cover smear with solution 1, allow it to act for 4 min.
- Rinse gently with distilled water and apply solution 2.
- Apply heat until steam forms (or about 50°C for 3 min) and allow solution 2 to remain on slide for 4 min.
- Rinse slide gently with distilled water.
- Allow it to air dry, and observe under oil immersion lens (100X).

Observations

Flagella appear dark in colour.
- Grey stain.
- Staining reagents.

GREY STAIN

i. Solution A—Mordant

Saturated aqueous solution of potassium alum	5 ml
Aqueous tannic acid (20%)	2 ml
Saturated aqueous solution of mercuric chloride	2 ml

- Mix and store.

ii. Solution B—Stain

Basic fuchsin (1% in distilled water)	10 ml
Methyl alcohol	10 ml

- Mix and store.

Staining Procedure

- Prepare a smear on clean glass slide and allow it to air dry.
- Apply solution A for 5–10 min.
- Wash with distilled water.
- Apply solution B for 5–10 min.
- Wash with tap water.
- Drain and dry.
- Observe under oil immersion lens (100X).

Observation

Flagella appear red in colour.

WET-MOUNT FLAGELLAR STAIN

Staining Reagents

i. Mordant Solution

Phenol (5% aqueous solution)	10 ml
Tannic acid	2 gm
Saturated aqueous solution of aluminium potassium sulphate	10 ml

ii. Ryu's Stain

Saturated ethanolic crystal violet	10 ml
Mordant solution	100 ml

- Filter stain and keep in a syringe with a 0.22 μm pore-size porus membrane between the syringe and needle.
- The needle is stuck in a rubber stopper to prevent drying.
- The stain remains stable for several weeks at ambient temperature.

Procedure

- Grow bacteria on blood agar or tryptic soy agar for 16–24 hrs.
- Take a loopful of water and touch onto the edge of a colony, and let motile bacteria swim into it.
- Transfer the loopful into a loopful of water on a clean glass slide.
- Place a clean cover-slip.
- Thus, bacterial suspension is prepared with minimum agitation to avoid detachment of flagella from cells.
- Allow this preparation to stand for 5–10 min, so that many bacterial cells attach to the surface of the slide and cover slip.
- Apply two drops of Ryu's stain to the edge of the cover slip and allow stain to diffuse into the film for 5–15 min.
- Observe under the microscope.

Observation

Flagella appear violet in colour.

Mechanism

The mordant and the silver nitrate form a deposit on the surface of flagella and thereby increase the thickness of flagella to such an extent that flagella can be made visible under the ordinary microscope.

14

Other Staining Methods

STAINING OF BACTERIAL CELL WALL

Chan's method is used for staining of bacterial cell wall (Fig. 14.1).

Staining Reagents
- Basic fuchsin
- Congo red

Procedure
- Prepare smear on a clean glass slide and allow it to air dry.
- Apply basic fuchsin and allow it to act for 2 min.
- Wash with water.
- Apply Congo red and allow it to act for 4 min.

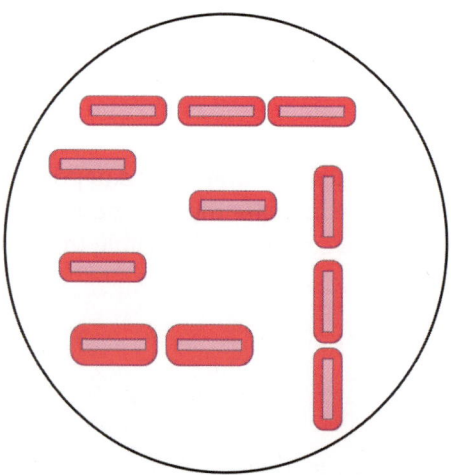

Fig. 14.1: Bacterial cell wall stained by Chan's method

- Wash with water and blot dry.
- Observe under oil immersion lens (100X).

Observations (Fig. 14.1)
- Cell wall appears dark pink in colour.
- Cytoplasm appears pink in colour.

STAINING OF NUCLEUS

Feulgen's method is used for staining of nucleus.

Staining Reagents
- 1N-hydrochloric acid solution
- Basic fuchsin

Procedure
- Prepare smear on a clean glass slide, allow it to dry and fix it by heat.
- Place the slide in 1N-hydrochloric acid solution for 10 min at 60°C in water bath.
- Wash slide with water.
- Apply basic fuchsin and allow it to react for 1 hour.
- Wash with water and blot dry.
- Observe under oil immersion lens (100X).

Observations
- Nucleus appears pink in colour
- Bacterial body appears colourless

STAINING OF PLAGUE BACILLI

Wayson stain is used to demonstrate bipolar staining characteristic of *Yersinia pestis,* in smears made from clinical material or rodent tissue, i.e. to demonstrate the characteristic safety pin appearance of plague bacilli (Fig. 14.2).

Staining Reagents

i. *Solution 1*

Basic fuchsin	0.3 gm
Absolute alcohol	8 ml

ii. *Solution 2*

Methylene blue	0.75 gm
Absolute alcohol	12 ml

- Mix solution 1 and 2.
- Add 5% phenol in distilled water and make it 200 ml by adding phenol solution.
- Mix it properly, boil and stand for 48 hours.
- Store this preparation—its storage for 1–2 yrs, enhances its staining ability.

Procedure

- Prepare smear on a clean glass slide.
- Fix smear preferably with alcohol or by heat.
- Apply Wayson stain and allow it to act for 7 min.
- Wash thoroughly with tap water.

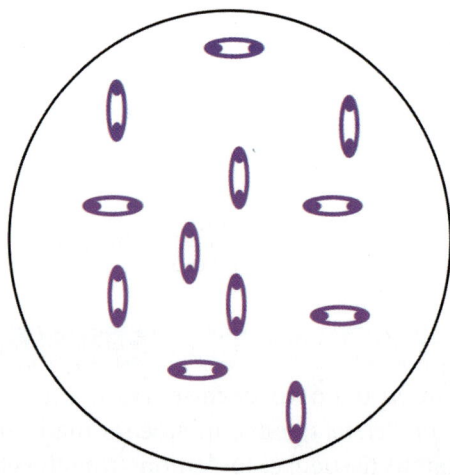

Fig. 14.2: Wayson stain showing safety pin appearance

- Allow it to dry in air.
- Observe smear under oil immersion lens (100X).

Observations

- *Y. pestis* appears purple in colour with a characteristic safety pin appearance (Fig. 14.2).
- It shows bipolar staining with two ends stained purple in colour with a central clear area.

Uses

- As stated above, it is used for diagnosis of plague.
- It can also be used for diagnosis of melioidosis.
- Also used as an alternative to detect *Y. enterocolitica*.

McFADYEAN'S METHOD

It is staining reaction used for presumptive diagnosis of anthrax.

Staining Reagent

Gurr's polychrome methylene blue as used in simple staining.

Procedure

- Prepare a thick smear on clean glass slide of blood, exudates or tissue fluid.
- Allow it to air dry and then fix it imperfectly by passing quickly through a flame for three times.
- Apply Gurr's polychrome methylene blue stain and allow it to act for 30 seconds.
- Wash with water and dry.
- Observe under oil immersion lens (100X).

Observation

Bacilli are stained blue in colour and are surrounded by irregular red-purple capsular material.

DIENES' STAIN

- Devised by Dienes' in 1939 and modified by Madoff in 1959.

- It is a staining method used for examination of colonies of mycoplasma grown on enriched media.

Staining Reagents

Azure II	0.25 gm
Methylene blue	0.5 gm
Maltose	2 gm
Na_2CO_3	0.05 gm
Benzoic acid	0.04 gm
Distilled water	20 ml

- Dissolve and filter before use.

Procedure

- The growth on agar plate or a portion of the plate is flooded with Dienes' stain diluted in 1 in 10 in distilled water.
- The plate is observed under a low-power objective lens (10X).

Alternatively

- Smear clean cover slips with the undiluted Dienes' stain.
- Allow it to dry.
- Cut a block of agar containing the colony from plate.
- Place agar block on microscopic slide.
- Cover this block with cover slip with dry stain.
- Observe this stained preparation under low power objective (10X).

Observations

- Colonies of *Mycoplasma*—stain intense royal blue.
- Colonies of *Ureaplasma*—stain reddish or greenish blue.

Note: Colonies of mycoplasma retain the stain for at least 2 days, while colonies of other bacteria lose colour in 30 min.

- Colonies of *Mycoplasma* are transferred to slides by the hot water transfer method.
- These colonies may be stained by overnight exposure to Dienes' stain or a mixture of Dienes' and Giemsa in equal proportions, and stained preparation may be viewed under oil immersion objective lens (100X).

CRESYL-FAST VIOLET STAIN

Devise by Shepard in 1967.

Staining Reagents

Cresyl-fast violet	1 gm
Distilled water (pH 3.7)	100 ml

- Adjust pH of distilled water to 3.7 by adding 1–5 drops of glacial acetic acid to 100 ml of distilled water.
- Dissolve 1 gm of cresyl-fast violet in 100 ml of distilled water.
- Allow solution to ripen for 48 hrs.
- This is used for preparation of working solution which is to be prepared daily.

Working Solution

Stock solution	20 ml
NaCl	0.05 gm

- Agitate for 1 min, filter and add 7 gm of maltose to it.

Procedure

- Same procedure as in Dienes' stain can be used, or
- Agar block is stained and then cover slip is applied.

Observation

Colonies of both *Mycoplasma* and *Ureaplasma* appear red-purple in colour.

GIEMSA STAIN

Procedure

- Blocks of agar containing colonies are cut and inverted on glass slides, and then immersed in Bouin's fixative overnight.
- The block is remove and slide is rinsed in tap water for 1 hour.
- The slide is placed in Petri dish with colony-side down on two supports.
- Giemsa stain diluted 1 in 20 in distilled water is added to Petri dish.

- Giemsa stain is allowed to act for overnight.
- Slide is rinsed and observed under microscope.

GIMENEZ STAIN

It is used to detect and identify bacterial infections in tissue, especially those infections caused by certain slow-growing or fastidious bacteria.

Staining Reagents

i. *Carbol Fuchsin Stock*

Phenol	2.5 ml
Absolute alcohol	5 ml
Basic fuchsin	0.5 gm
Distilled water	50 ml

- Can be stored at room temperature for 1 year.

ii. *Sodium Phosphate Buffer pH 7.5*

iii. *Malachite Green*

- Gimenez stain is prepared by mixing 4 ml of carbol fuchsin stock solution with 10 ml of sodium phosphate buffer (pH 7.5).
- This stain remains stable for 48 hours at 4°C.
- It is to be filtered before use.

Procedure

- Prepare a smear on a clean glass slide, allow it to dry in air and then fix it by heat.
- Cover smear with Gimenez stain and allow it to act for 2–3 minutes.
- Wash with water.
- Apply malachite green—a counter stain and allow it to act for 2–3 minutes.
- Wash with water, allow slide to dry in air and observe under oil immersion lens (100X).

Observations

- Rickettsia appear bright red in colour.
- Background appears blue-green in colour.

MACHIAVELLO'S STAIN (MODIFIED)

It is used to demonstrate rickettsia in tissue sections.

Staining Reagents

i. Methylene Blue (1%)

Methylene blue	1 gm
Distilled water	100 ml

- Can be stored at room temperature for 3 months.

ii. Basic Fuchsin (0.25%)

Basic fuchsin	0.25 gm
Distilled water	100 ml

- Can be stored at room temperature for one month.

iii. Citric Acid (0.5%)

Citric acid	0.5 gm
Distilled water	95 ml

- Can be stored at room temperature for 2 months.

Procedure

- Cut paraffin sections of 4–5 μ.
- Deparaffinize and hydrate to distilled water.
- Apply methylene blue solution and allow it to act for overnight.
- Decolourize in 95% alcohol.
- Apply counter stain (0.25% basic fuchsin) and allow it to act for 30 min.
- Decolourize rapidly with citric acid solution for 1 or 2 seconds and not more than 3 seconds.
- Differentiate rapidly in absolute alcohol.
- Dehydrate in 95% alcohol and absolute alcohol—3 changes each.

- Clear in xylene—3 changes.
- Mount with permount and observe.

Observations

- Rickettsia are stained bright red in colour.
- Nuclei are stained blue in colour.

RICE METHOD OF STAINING (MODIFIED)

It is used for staining the inclusion bodies of trachoma and inclusion conjunctivitis.

Staining Reagent

Lugol's iodine: 5% iodine in 10% potassium iodide.

Procedure

- Smear scrapings on clean dry slides and allow to dry in air for at least 5 min.
- Cover slide with Lugol's iodine.
- Allow it to act for 2 min or more (if required in case of dry specimens).
- Care should be taken to avoid drying and crystallization of the stain on the slide.
- Wash with water.
- Blot dry and observe under oil immersion lens (100X).

Observations

- Inclusions are stained—deep orange-brown in colour.
- Background—golden yellow.

15

Fluorochrome Staining

INTRODUCTION

- Fluorochrome staining using fluorochrome dyes such as auramine O and rhodamine are fluorescent staining methods that can be used for demonstration of acid-fast bacilli.
- The organisms stained with fluorescent dyes become self-luminous and are seen as bright objects against a dark background.
- Auramine–phenol fluorochrome staining technique can be used an alternative method for Ziehl-Neelsen staining method for demonstration of *Mycobacterium tuberculosis* in sputum, CSF and other specimens.
- Fluorochrome staining is more sensitive than Ziehl-Neelsen staining method technique for detection of mycobacteria.

Staining Reagents

i. *Auramine O Stain*

Auramine O	3 gm
Phenol	30 gm
Distilled water	1000 ml

- Dissolve the phenol in water with gentle heat.
- Add the auramine gradually and shake vigorously until dissolved.
- Filter and store in a dark-stoppered bottle.

ii. *Decolourizing Solution*

75% (v/v) industrial alcohol (ethanol) in water containing 0.5% NaCl and 0.5% HCl.

iii. *Potassium Permanganate Solution (Counter Stain)*

$KMnO_4$	1 gm
Distilled water	1000 ml

- Dissolve potassium permanganate in distilled water.
- Store in brown bottle. Or

Iv. *Acridine Orange Solution (Counter Stain)*

Dibasic sodium phosphate	0.01 gm
Distilled water	100 ml
Acridine orange	0.01 gm

- Dissolve sodium phosphate in distilled water.
- Add acridine orange and dissolve it properly.
- Store in tightly stoppered or closed brown bottle.

Procedure

- Prepare a thin smear of sputum or other specimen on a clean glass slide.
- Fix it by flaming.
- Cover smear with the auramine O solution and allow it to act for 15 minutes at room temperature. Do not heat the smear.
- Wash with tap water. If tap water is not clean, use filtered or clean boiled rain water for washing the smear.
- Apply the acid—alcohol decolourizing solution and allow it to act for 5 minutes.
- Wash off the decolourizer with water from the tap, rinse well.
- Cover the slide with potassium permanganate solution or acridine orange solution for 1–2 minutes but not more than four minutes.
- Wash well with tap water.
- Allow to air dry, do not use blotting paper.
- To prevent fading of the fluorescence, protect the stained smear from sunlight and bright light and observe within 24 hours.
- Observe the smear as soon as possible (within a few hours) under fluorescence microscope–initially under 10X objective

to focus the smear and then observe systematically under 40X objective for AFB.

• Immediate observation of smear is important, as fading of the fluorescence occurs with time.

Observations

• AFB appears bright yellow colour rods of variable in length, often curved or fragmented
• Background appears dark in colour.

Grading of Sputum Smear

The smear is graded as follows (IUATLD/WHO system)—using 40X objective, 10X objective (Table 15.1).

Table 15.1: Grading of smear

No. of AFB	Seen in (number of fields)	Report
00	40	No AFB seen
1–9	40	Scanty AFB
20–199	40	1+
5–50	Per field (examine 20 fields)	2+
>50	Per field (examine 8 fields)	3+

Note: When no AFB are seen after examining 40 fields, report the smear as 'no AFB seen'. A second sputum specimen should be examined.

MODIFICATIONS OF FLUOROCHROME STAINING

Two different modifications include:

1. Richards-Miller fluorescence microscopy
2. Silver-Sonnenwirth-Alex modification.

Richards-Miller Fluorescence Microscopy

Procedure

• Decontaminate and concentrate the clinical specimen by using suitable concentration method.
• Prepare smear on a clean glass slide and fix in usual manner.

- Apply and stain smears for 4–5 minutes in 0.1% aqueous solution of fluorescent dye auramine O, to which 3% liquid phenol has been added.
- Rinse with water.
- Decolourize smear for 4–5 minute in 70% ethyl alcohol containing 0.5% HCl and 0.5 % NaCl.
- Rinse in water again.
- Allow to dry in air. Do not blot dry the smear.
- Observe under fluorescent microscope—initially under high dry magnification and verify with oil immersion objective.

Observations

Acid-fast bacilli fluoresce with a characteristics golden glow against a dark background.

Silver-Sonnenwirth-Alex Modification

This is another modification used for demonstration of mycobacteria.

Staining Reagents

i. *Auramine Rhodamine stain*

Auramine O	1.5 gm
Rhodamine B	0.75 gm
Glycerol	75 ml
Phenol crystals liquefied at 50°C	10 ml
Distilled water	50 ml

- Keep stock solution at room temperature and filter before use through Whatman no. 2 filter paper.

ii. *Decolourizer*

HCl	0.5 ml
Ethyl alcohol, 70%	99.5 ml
NaCl	0.5 g

iii. *Counter stain*

Potassium permanganate	0.5 g
Distilled water	100 ml

Procedure

- Prepare smear on a clean glass slide from clinical specimen.
- Allow it to air dry and fix it by heating using a Bunsen burner.
- Cover smear with auramine rhodamine stain and allow it to act at 37°C for 30 minutes.
- Decolourize smear for 10 minutes with acid–alcohol decolourizer.
- Apply counter stain and allow it to act for 2 minutes.

Procedure for Tissues

- Tissues that have been deparaffinized by washing in 3 changes of xylene for 1.5 minute and hydrated by dipping in absolute alcohol, 95% alcohol, 10% alcohol and water can be stained with staining reagents mentioned above.
- Staining should be done in stain preheated to 60°C.
- Slides should be immersed in preheated stain for 10 minute and slide should be kept at 60°C in incubator.
- After primary staining procedure is completed, wash slide for 2 minutes.
- Decolourize smear with 0.5% HCl in ethyl alcohol for 2–3 minutes.
- Rinse smear in tap water for 2 minutes.
- Apply counter stain and allow it to act for 1 minute.
- Wash in water for 2 minutes.
- Blot dry the smear.
- Dehydrate smear for 15 seconds in absolute alcohol.
- Dip slide in xylol for clearing.
- Mount smear in DPX mount.
- Observe smear under fluorescent microscope.

Observations

Mycobacterium tuberculosis and atypical mycobacteria fluoresce a reddish, golden yellow against a black background.

Advantages of Fluorochrome Staining

- Using a fluorochrome staining technique, a smear can be examined at lower magnification, and thus, it allows examination of more area in a shorter time; hence, less fields are required to be examined.

- When AFBs are a few in number, can be easily seen by flurochrome staining and they are more likely to be detected in a fluorochrome stained smear.
- With the recent development of light emitting diode (LED), it is now possible to examine smears inexpensively and easily by fluorescence microscopy.
- Auramine fluoresces when illuminated (excited) by blue violet or ultraviolet (UV) light. It can be used to demonstrate AFB because it binds to the mycolic acid in the bacterial cell wall.
- No heating is required as in ZN staining. After they are stained with auramine, the smear is decolorized with acid alcohol, which removes the dye from the background. The smear is then washed with a weak solution of potassium permanganate to darken the background. Tubercle bacilli fluoresce bright yellow against a dark (permanganate) or orange (acridine orange) background.

ACRIDINE ORANGE STAIN FOR CHROMIDIAL BARS

The acridine orange can be used to visualize chromidial bars of *Entamoeba coli, Entamoeba histolytica/E. dispar* and *Entamoeba hartmanni*.

Staining Reagent

Acridine Orange (Acetate Buffered)

Acridine orange   1 ml
Glacial acetic acid   0.5 ml
Buffered water pH 6.8   8.5 ml

Procedure

- Add an equal volume of stain to the concentrate.
- Observe the deposit under UV light after 30 minutes.

Observations

The chromidial bars fluoresce bright green in colour under UV microscope.

Auramine–Phenol Stain

Procedure

- Prepare faecal smears on clean glass slides as for ZN.
- Fix smear in methanol.
- Apply auramine–phenol and allow it to act for 10–15 min.
- Rinse thoroughly in tap water.
- Decolourise smear in acid alcohol (as for ZN).
- Rinse thoroughly in tap water.
- Apply counter stain—0.1% potassium permanganate for 30 seconds.
- Rinse thoroughly in tap water, allow to air dry. Do not blot dry to avoid false positive fluorescence of blotting paper.
- Observe under UV microscope.

Observations

Oocysts of cryptosporidia appear as bright yellow discs against a dark background.

16

Immunofluorescence Staining

- Fluorescence is the property of absorbing the light rays of one particular wavelength and emitting the light rays of a different wavelength.
- Fluorescent dyes can absorb ultraviolet (UV) light and can convert/reflect back them into visible light.
- This reflected light is visualized by a fluorescent microscope under ultraviolet radiation.
- Fluorescent dyes (fluorochromes) such as fluorescein isothiocyanate, tetramethyl rhodamine, dansyl and phycoerythrin can be used to detect infected cells in exudates, secretions and tissues.
- Fluorescein isothiocyanate is the most commonly used. It emits a greenish/yellow light.
- Rhodamine emits red/orange light and dansyl emits yellow light.

Types

Two types:

1. *Direct immunofluorescence* is used for detection of microbes.
2. *Indirect immunofluorescence* is used for detection of antibodies (Abs).

Direct Immunofluorescence

- In this, the fluorochrome can be conjugated to Abs and used to locate and identify antigens (Ags) in specimens.
- By applying a known antiserum (Abs) labelled with fluorochrome to smear of specimen fixed on a glass slide, it

is possible to detect infected cells in specimen by locating the Ag.

Requirements

i. Specific Abs raised against the Ag to be detected.
ii. Fluorescent dye—fluorescein isothiocyanate is most commonly used. The fluorescent dye is to be conjugated with IgG Abs.
iii. Acetone
iv. Phosphate buffered saline (pH 7.2).
v. Buffered glycerol (pH 7.2).
vi. 10% glycerol in PBS.
vii. Counter stain—diluted Evan's blue (1 µg/ml) or ethidium bromide (0.5 µg/ml) in PBS.
viii. Bovine serum albumin.

Procedure

• Prepare a smear on a clean glass slide from a clinical specimen or broth culture of organism.
• Allow it to air dry.
• Fix smear in cold acetone (at 4°C) for 5 minutes. Alternatively, smear can be fixed by using alcohol.
• Apply a drop of fluorescein labeled Ab solution to smear and allow it to spread gently over the surface of smear.
• Allow this conjugate to act for 30 minutes at 37°C.
• Wash slide twice in PBS—two 5 minutes washes.
• Blot dry the slide.
• Add one drop of 90% glycerol—PBS (buffered glycerol) and cover with a cover-slip.
• Addition of 1–10 µg/ml of para—phenylenediamine to the mounting medium (i.e. buffered glycerol) is recommended to prevent the fading of fluorescence.
• 0.1–0.25 M n-propyl gallate can be used instead of para-phenylenediamine as an anti-fading agent to delay the process of fading.
• After mounting observe smear under fluorescent microscope for the presence or absence of the fluorescence.

Observations (Fig. 16.1)

- Fluorescence under UV microscope is considered as positive.
- Green fluorescence is observed.
- No fluorescence under UV microscope is considered as negative.

Counter Staining

- Smears stained with fluorescein isothiocyanate may be counterstained with Evan's blue or ethidium bromide.
- This helps in outlining the cell morphology and permits an evaluation of the proportion of cells which stain positive with fluorescent dye–Ab conjugate.

Uses

- Commonly used for detection of different bacteria, viruses, fungi and parasites in tissues, blood, CSF, urine, faeces and other fluids.
- Also used for detection of other Ags such as tumour Ags, organ and tissue Ags, blood cells, enzymes, hormones, etc.
- It is most commonly used in the diagnosis of viral infections such as rabies, measles, mumps, etc.

Advantages

- It is more sensitive for detection and localization of microbial Ags in specimens.
- It is specific also, and it is more specific when fluorochrome is labeled with monoclonal Abs.
- It is a rapid method.
- It useful for identification of viruses also.

Disadvantages

- Quantitation is difficult.
- It requires UV radiation for visualization.
- It requires expertise personnel for reporting.
- There is a chance of fading of stain.
- It may give false positive results.
- It require expensive equipment.

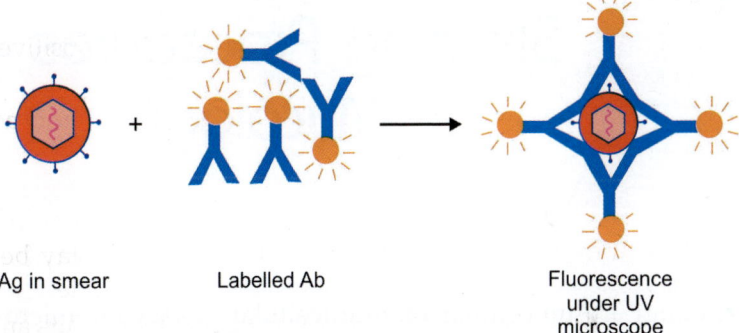

| Ag in smear | Labelled Ab | Fluorescence under UV microscope |

Fig. 16.1: Direct immunofluorescence stain

Mechanism

- In this method specific Abs raised against the Ag (microbe) to be detected is conjugated with a fluorescent dye.
- The conjugate of fluorescent dye—Ab is used to detect unknown Ag (microbe) in the specimen.
- If Ag (microbe) is present in the specimen, it will bind with the conjugate.
- When observed under the fluorescent microscope using ultra-violet radiations, the conjugate of fluorescent dye—Ab bound to Ag (microbe) emits a fluorescence (Fig. 16.1).

17

Staining Procedures in Mycology

- Fungi are unicellular or multicellular eukaryotic micro-organisms causing a variety of diseases in human beings.
- They are now recognized as significant causes of morbidity and mortality.
- The incidence of fungal diseases has increased in recent past because of underlying predisposing factors.
- Direct microscopic examination is the most important part in the laboratory diagnosis of fungal infections. It helps in rapid diagnosis of fungal infections.
- Different staining methods used in the diagnosis of fungal infections include the following.

WET PREPARATIONS

The wet preparations are used for direct demonstration of fungal elements in the clinical specimens or to study morphological features of fungal isolate. Different wet preparations used are as follows.

1. Potassium Hydroxide Mounts

Principle

- The aqueous potassium hydroxide (KOH) digests protein debris and dissolves cement substance, which holds keratinized cells together.
- KOH thus helps to clear the structures which may be confused with fungal elements.
- The addition of 10% glycerol decreases precipitation of KOH in reagent bottles and allows the KOH preparation to be kept for 18 hours or longer.

Reagents

Potassium hydroxide	10 gm
Glycerol	10 ml
Distilled water	80 ml

- The addition of glycerol helps to prevent drying.
- The concentration of KOH can be increased depending upon nature of clinical material, as solid specimens require 10–40% concentration.
- Dimethyl sulfoxide (DMSO) can be added to 20% KOH solution. It acts as cleansing agent. This reagent contains:

KOH	20 gm
DMSO	40 ml
Distilled water	60 ml

Procedure

- Two different procedures of KOH mount can be used.
- These include slide KOH and tube KOH.

i. Slide KOH

- Place a drop of 10% KOH in the center of a clean glass slide.
- Place epidermal scales, skin scrapings, nail clippings or homogenized biopsy tissue in KOH, and tease apart with the help of teasing needles to produce a thin KOH preparation.
- Cover preparation with a cover slip, gently heat the slide by passing it through a Bunsen burner flame for 3–4 times.
- Do not overheat the slide otherwise crystals of KOH will be formed.
- If specimen is not properly dissolved, it may be kept for some more time in a wet Petri dish and observed.
- If DMSO is used, heating is not required.
- A mixture of 20% KOH solution and equal part of Parker ink may also be used for staining fungal elements.
- A drop of 0.01% acridine orange may be added to KOH slide and is observed under fluorescent microscope.

- Observe the preparation using the low power (10X) objective of the microscope and then under the high dry (45/47X) objective to confirm observations.

ii. *Tube KOH*

- The tube KOH preparation is used mainly for biopsy specimens, which take longer time for dissolution.
- This procedure is also adapted in case of nail clippings and skin biopsy, which also dissolve with difficulty. These specimens may need increased concentration of KOH.
- The homogenized biopsy tissue is dissolved in 10% KOH and examined after keeping for an overnight in an incubator at 37°C.

Observations

- If any fungal elements are seen report it as positive and mention the structure of fungi seen.
- Fungi may show different morphological forms, e.g.:
  - Yeast cells
  - Budding cells
  - Pseudohyphae
  - True hyphae
  - Septate hyphae
  - Aseptate hyphae, etc.
- The positive findings are reported according to the structure seen, e.g.:
  - Positive for yeast cells, or
  - Positive for true hyphae.
- If no fungal elements are seen, report it as "**No fungal elements**" are seen.

2. Saline Wet Mount

Principle

Saline mount is used to observe clinical specimens and pure cultures of yeasts.

Reagent

Sterile normal saline.

Procedure (Fig. 17.1)

- Place a small drop of saline on a clean, glass slide.
- Suspend a small amount of clinical specimen or culture in the saline.
- Gently cover slip the preparation.
- Observe under low power and high power objectives for the presence of the fungal elements.

India Ink Stain

It is used as a negative stain for demonstration of capsulated yeasts.

Principle

The capsule on yeast cells repels the carbon particles in India ink that results in a clear, capsular "halo" around cells.

Staining Reagents

India ink	150 ml
Merthiolate ink (1:1000)	3 ml
Tween 80 (1:10,000)	0.1 ml

- Mix, filter and keep in dropping bottle.

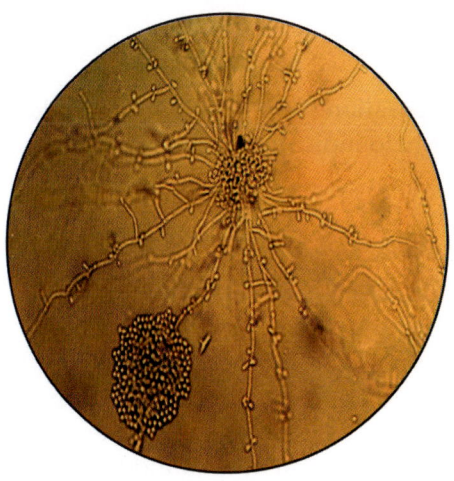

Fig. 17.1: Fungal elements in wet mount

- India ink is easily contaminated with bacteria, yeast, or fungal spores; hence, the reagent should be checked periodically for contamination with these cells by preparing a mount without adding specimen and should be filtered periodically to remove bacterial contamination and carbon particles. If correctly prepared one should be able to barely read newsprint through the preparation.

Procedure

- Place two or three loopfuls (one small drop) of diluted India ink in the center of a clean-glass slide.
- Add a drop of the specimen to be studied (body fluids, urine, CSF, etc.). Tissue should be homogenized before using. Only a small portion should be used if working with an unknown yeast colony.
- Mix well. Preparation should be brownish, not black, in color. It may be diluted with sterile distilled water, if necessary, and should be covered with a coverslip. Care should be taken not to trap bubbles in the preparation.
- Blot dry the excess fluid.
- Observe the preparation using the low power (10X) objective of a microscope and then under high dry (45/47X) objective to confirm observations.

Observations

- Positive preparation shows presence of budding yeast cells with a clear halo indicative of capsular material (Fig. 17.2).
- Negative preparation shows no yeast cells or yeast cells without the halo.

Modified India Ink Staining

- India ink staining technique may be modified by adding 2% chromium mercury.
- In the modified method, a drop of CSF is placed on a clean glass slide to which 2% chromium mercury is added and mixed well. Then a small drop of India ink is added to it and cover slip is placed.

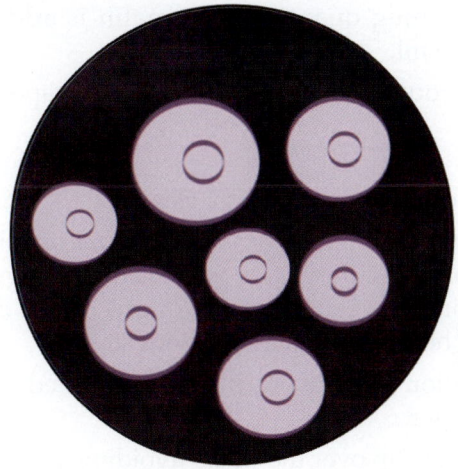

Fig. 17.2: India ink preparation showing capsulated round yeast cells of *Cryptococcus neoformans*

- The preparation is observed under bright-field microscope.
- This helps observation of external and internal structures of organism.

Nigrosin Stain

Principle

- Nigrosin staining is also negative staining technique can be used as an alternative to India ink stain to determine an organism's cellular morphology.
- It is also a background staining method that stains the background whereas the organism remains unstained and the morphology is not distorted in any way.
- Capsules displace the dye and appear as halos surrounding the organism.

Staining Reagents

Nigrosin granules   10 gm
Formalin (10%)   100 ml

- Nigrosin is to be added to 25 ml of formalin and boiled in water bath for 30 minutes.

- Then remaining quantity of formalin is added to make volume 100 ml.
- Filtered through double Whatmann filter paper no. 1.

Procedure

- Place a drop of nigrosin onto a clean glass slide.
- Add 1 drop of specimen or liquid culture or rub a speck of material on the slide surface just beside the nigrosin before mixing it into the stain. Sputum or pus can be cleared with KOH and heat and then mixed with stain.
- If preparation is too dark, it may be diluted with a small drop of water.
- Place a cover slip over the smear avoiding air bubbles, press it down gently through a sheet of blotting paper so that the film becomes very thin and pale in colour.
- Observe under high power objective of phase-contrast microscope for the presence of encapsulated cells.
- Nigrosin stain can be used as an alternative to India ink stain. This is better than India ink stain as it can last for more than one year and no carbon particles appear in staining solution.
- India ink is free from antimicrobial agents and hence, there is risk of getting infection while handling the stain. This is not possible with nigrosin which contains formalin.

Observations

- Organisms possessing a capsule appear highly refractile, surrounded by a clear zone or halo against a dark background.
- Leukocytes may also appear haloed due to leakage of the cytoplasm but the halo has a fuzzy, irregular appearance at the periphery and the cell within the halo has a paler cell wall.
- Some *Cryptococcus neoformans* strains have been reported to be nigrosin stain negative.
- No clear zone around the organism is considered as negative.

Quality Control Organisms

- **Positive control:** *Coccus neoformans* or other capsulate organisms.
- **Negative control:** A proven negative smear may be used as the negative control. *Candida albicans* could be used as it is non-encapsulated.

Calcofluor White Stain

Principle

- Calcofluor white (CFW) is water-soluble, non-toxic, colorless textile dye and fluorescent brightener.
- It selectively binds to cellulose and chitin present in the fungal cell wall and visualized when exposed to long wavelength ultraviolet and short wavelength visible light.

Staining Reagents

i. *Solution A*

Calcofluor white	1.9 gm
Distilled water	100 ml

- The calcofluor solution is prepared by dissolving calcoflour white powder in distilled water.

ii. *Solution B*

Evans' blue	0.05 gm
Distilled water	100 ml

Working Solution

- 1 ml of solution A is mixed with 9 ml of solution B.
- Mix well and store in refrigerator.
- Evans' blue solution is added in order to reduce non-specific background fluorescence and reveal surrounding tissue.
- Evans' blue is a counter stain, which also produces contrasting orange to ruby-red background thereby enhancing detection of fungi.

Procedure

- Place a portion of the specimen on the slide (select a purulent area of secretions).

- Add 1 to 2 drops of KOH and emulsify specimen. If it does not clear rapidly, place slide in Petri dish and allow it to stand for about 10 minutes.
- If tissues or scrapings, place the slide on 35°C bench top heating block for 15–20 minutes to speed clearing.
- Apply 1 or 2 drops of calcofluor white reagent and mix thoroughly. Calcofluor white may be added right after KOH.
- Apply cover slip gently. Make sure that specimen does not overflow.
- Observe under fluorescent microscope.
- Always use a control slide positive for yeast or filamentous fungus.
- Calcofluor white aqueous solution shows absorption over the range of 300 to 412 nm, with an absorbance peak at 347 nm. This means that maximum excitation and fluorescence occurs with ultraviolet light, although excitation with violet or blue violet light also gives good results.

Observations

- Fungi, cysts of *Pneumocystis carinii* and other parasites stained with calcofluor white display a brilliant apple-green fluorescence under ultraviolet light and violet under blue light.
- Yellowish-green background fluorescence may be observed with tissue samples.
- The fluorescence displayed by fungal or parasitic structures is much more intense and highly visible.
- Background fluorescence can be diminished by examining slides under blue light or by using various exciter and barrier filter combinations.
- Yeast cells can be differentiated from *P. carinii* by budding and deep internal staining.
- Cotton fibers will fluoresce strongly and must be differentiated from fungal hyphae.
- Background fluorescence may be present but fungi exhibit a more intense fluorescence.

- Amoebic cysts fluorescent but trophozoites are not stained and do not show fluorescence.
  - **Positive control:** *Candida albicans* shows fluorescence
  - **Negative control:** *Escherichia coli* shows no fluorescence or shows weak fluorescence.

Advantage

It is more sensitive method for demonstration of fungi as compared to other methods commonly used.

> For detection of fungi in clinical specimens calcofluor white stain is superior to conventional staining techniques. It is technically simple, quick and highly reliable to identify fungi even if observer is relatively inexperienced.

Lactophenol Cotton Blue Stain

Principle

- Cotton blue (China blue) stains chitin and cellulose. As fungal cell walls are rich in chitin, this stain is an excellent choice for observing fungi in clinical specimens.
- LCB is of two types:
  - Plain LCB
  - LCB with polyvinyl alcohol

Staining Reagents

i. *Plain LCB*

Melted phenol crystals	20 ml
Lactic acid	20 ml
Glycerol	40 ml
Cotton blue	0.050 or 0.075 gm
Distilled water	20 ml

- Mix well all the reagents properly and dissolve 0.050 gm or 0.075 gm of cotton blue stain in distilled water before mixing with remaining reagents.
- In this preparation used for examination of fungi
  - Phenol acts as disinfectant
  - Lactic acid preserves morphology of fungi

– Glycerol is hygroscopic agent—prevents drying
– Cotton blue stains outer wall of fungus.

ii. *LCB with polyvinyl alcohol*

Polyvinyl alcohol (PVA) powder   15 gm
Distilled water   100 ml

- Mix PVA powder at 80°C in a beaker placed in a water bath.
- A thick viscous solution is formed and if this mixture is lumpy.
- Filter it through double-layered cloth.

Staining Solution

PVA stock solution   56 ml
Melted phenol   22 ml
Lactic acid   22 ml
Cotton blue   0.05 gm

- Add lactic acid to polyvinyl alcohol stock solution, mix it well and then add phenol.
- Mix and warm gently to dissolve.
- This LCB preparation prepared using PVA can be permanently preserved.

Procedure

i. *Tease mount preparation*

- Place a small drop of lactophenol cotton blue (LCB) in the center of a clean glass slide.
- Remove a small fragment of fungus colony and the supporting agar at a point between the center and periphery and place in the LCB.
- With the help of needle gently tease apart the fungus culture first and then spread it in the LCB.
- Place the cover slip. Do not press or tap the cover slip because this tends to break the conidia from the conidiophores and make identification more difficult, or impossible.
- For appropriate staining, allow stain to act for longer duration around 30 min.

- The preparation may be preserved indefinitely by sealing the edges with colored nail polish after wiping off excess mounting medium. Colored polish has been found to last longer than clear polish.
- Observe the preparation using the low power (10X) objective of a microscope. Use a high dry (45/47X) objective to confirm observations.

Observation (Fig. 17.3)
- Fungal elements—yeast cells, mycelia and fruiting structures appear blue in colour.
- The background appears a faint, pale blue in colour.
- The absence of fungal elements indicates a negative result.

Quality control organisms
- *Positive control:* A proven positive specimen may be used as the positive control.
- *Negative control:* A proven negative specimen may be used as the negative control.

ii. *Needle-mount method*
- Place a drop of 95% alcohol on a clean glass slide.
- Take a small portion of culture in the alcohol and tease out it with the help of needles or straight wires.
- Spread it properly and allow alcohol to evaporate then add a drop of LCB stain.

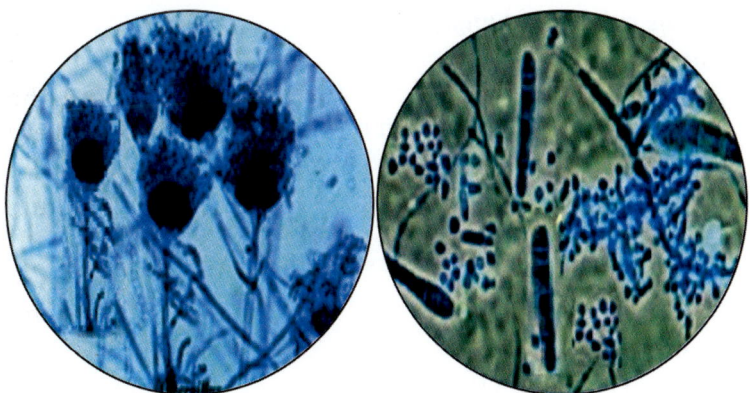

Fig. 17.3: LCB mount of fungi under high power (40X)

- Apply cover slip, avoid bubbles and press it.
- Remove excess stain around the cover slip with the help of blotting paper.
- Allow stain to penetrate for a few minutes.
- Observe this preparation under 10X and 40X .
- The edges of cover slip can be sealed with nail varnish or cellulose lacquer and the preparation can be preserved permanently.

Observations
- Fungal elements appear blue in colour.
- Background appears faint, pale blue in colour.

iii. *Scotch tape preparation*
- Place a drop of LCB on a clean glass slide.
- Touch the adhesive side of the transparent scotch tape to the surface of the colony on agar plate at a point immediate between the center and periphery of the colony.
- Place and fix the adhesive side of the scotch tape over an area on the glass slide containing LCB.
- Observe the preparation under 10X and 40X.

Observations
- Fungal elements appear dark blue in colour.
- Background appears faint, pale blue in colour.

iv. *Slide culture technique*
Principle
- Conidia formed by fungi play an important role in accurate identification of some fungi but sometimes, conidia from a culture may not be observed in a Lactophenol Cotton Blue preparation because of teasing of growth.
- Slide culture technique helps in accurate identification by allowing periodic observation of intact growth of fungi and their conidia without disturbing their morphology.

Requirements
- Sterile Petri plate (15 × 100 mm).
- Filter paper (100 mm diameter).

- Sterile distilled water.
- Sterile pipettes.
- Sterile scalpel.
- Sabouraud's dextrose agar, potato dextrose agar (PDA) or other suitable medium in a Petri plate.
- Sterile microscopic glass slides and cover slips.

Procedure
- With the help of sterile scalpel cut one square cm blocks of agar from agar plate.
- With the help of flat side of scalpel, transfer agar block to center of sterile slide.
- Place a piece of filter paper in the bottom of a sterile Petri dish.
- With a sterile probe, inoculate the edges of the agar in 3 or 4 areas with small fragments of the fungal colony.
- With the help of sterile forceps place a sterile cover slip on the agar block.
- Thoroughly moisten the filter paper by placing approximately 1.5 ml of sterile distilled water along the edge of the Petri dish and allowing the filter paper to absorb it.
- Incubate the culture at room temperature.
- When growth appears beneath the cover slip remove the slide culture from the Petri plate and dry the bottom of the slide.
- Gently lift cover slip from agar block with the help of pair of sterile forceps and place a drop of LCB and place the cover slip removed from the agar block on the LCB.
- Observe the slide under low power (10X) and/or high dry (45/47X).

Observations
- Fungal elements appear dark blue in colour.
- Based on the type of hyphae, arrangement of conidiophores, morphology of conidia, etc. accurate identification of type of fungus is possible.

Pal, Hasegawa, Ono and Lee Stain (PHOL Stain)

- This staining method is devised by Pal, Hasegawa, Ono and Lee; hence, the name.
- This stain is used similar to LCB stain for examination of fungal isolates and *Prototheca* species.
- It contains formalin instead of phenol and methylene blue in place of cotton blue of lactophenol cotton blue stain.

Neutral Red Stain

- Neutral red staining is a vital staining method.
- It is used to find out the vitality/viability of fungi.
- It is the simplest method for evaluation of viability of fungal elements.
- Neutral red is a water-soluble dye that is capable of passing through intact plasma membrane and is stored in lysosomes of viable cells.
- When cell membrane and lysosomes are damaged, the uptake of neutral red ceases. Because of this property, it has been used as vital stain.

Diazonium Blue B Reagent (DBB Reagent)

- DBB reagent is used for differentiation of species of genera *Trichosporon* and *Geotrichum* spp.
- Alkali–ethanol DBB reaction is most reliable out of different types of procedures utilized for performing this color test showing red-stained colonies in basidiomycetes.
- Positive reaction is indicated if dark-red or violet red color develops within two minutes.
- *Trichosporon* isolates form pink to violet pigments following reaction with DBB that differentiates them from *Geotrichum* species which are DBB-negative.
- This modification facilitates use of DBB reaction in clinical laboratories. The molecular basis of DBB reaction is not known.
- The test represents reproducible and empirical method of differentiating yeasts with basidiomycetous affinity from yeast with ascomycetous affinity as colonies of Ascomycetes remain unstained.

- *Malassezia* species are also DBB-positive.
- The DBB-positive *Candida* species have been now re-designated to either *Cryptococcus* genus or *Rhodotorula* genus.
- Negative DBB reaction is also of paramount importance for identification of yeast-like fungi.

Differential Stain—Gram's Stain

- Gram's stain can be used for detection of some of the fungal pathogens.
- Brown and Brenn modification of Gram's stain is used.

Procedure

- Prepare a smear on a clean glass slide and allow it to dry in air.
- Fix smear by passing it over flame.
- Place 0.5% aqueous crystal violet or methyl violet solution on slide for 30–60 seconds.
- Wash smear gently in tap water.
- Apply Gram's iodine solution and allow it to act for 30–60 seconds.
- Wash with tap water.
- Decolorize with solution of equal parts of acetone and 95% ethanol and wash immediately in running tap water.
- Counter stain with 0.5% aqueous safranine for 10 seconds or with dilute carbol fuchsin for 30–60 seconds.
- Wash with tap water, air or blot dry.
- Observe under oil immersion lens (100X).

Observations (Fig. 17.4)

- Fungi appear Gram-positive—violet-colored structures in stained smear.
- The Gram reaction in fungi depends on the permeability of the fungal cell wall to the dye-iodine complex as in bacteria.

Differential Stain—Acid-fast Stain

Modified acid-fast (Kinyoun's) stain is used for staining of fungal elements, which are acid-fast in nature.

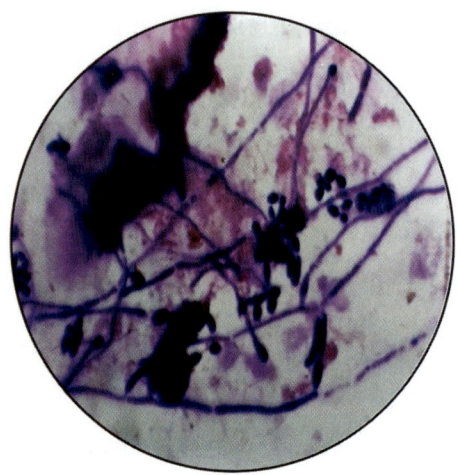

Fig. 17.4: Gram stained smear showing violet-coloured fungal elements

Staining Reagents

    i. *Kinyoun's carbol fuchsin*
       Basic fuchsin solution (3 gm basic
       fuchsin in 100 ml 95% ethyl alcohol)   10 ml
       Phenol (5% aqueous)   90 ml
   ii. *Decolourizer (1% sulfuric acid)*
       H_2SO_4 (concentrated)   1 ml
       Distilled water   99 ml
  iii. *Methylene blue*
       Methylene blue   0.3 gm
       Distilled water   100 ml

Procedure

- Prepare smear on a clean glass slide and fix the smear by gentle heating.
- Flood the smear with Kinyoun's carbol fuchsin solution.
- Allow the slide to stand for 20 minutes.
- Wash the smear with tap water.
- Decolorize the smear with 1% sulfuric acid until no more colour appears in the washing (approximately 1 min).

- Rinse with tap water.
- Counter stain with methylene blue for approximately 1 min.
- Rinse with tap water and air dry.

Observations

- The hat-shaped ascospores of *Pichia anomala* appear pink in colour
- Background appears blue in colour.

Hematoxylin and Eosin Stain

Principle

- It is a basic staining method used to stain nuclei in shade of blue by oxidized hematoxylin (hematin).
- Oxidized form of hematoxylin is weakly anionic purple stain, which has no particular affinity for nucleic acid of cell nuclei.
- It is combined with metallic salt or mordant with hematoxylin to confer net positive charge to the dye–mordant compound.
- The cationic dye–mordant/metal complex will bind to anionic nuclear chromatin.

Staining Reagents

i. **Hematoxylin stain**
   Cole's hematoxylin

Hematoxylin	3 gm
Ethyl alcohol	125 ml
Potassium or ammonium alum 160 gm	
Iodine	1 gm
Distilled water	2000 ml

ii. **Eosin 1% aqueous**

iii. **Differentiator**
   1% HCl in 70% alcohol

iv. **Blueing agent**
   Scott's tap water

Sodium bicarbonate	2 gm
Magnesium sulphate	20 gm
Water	2000 ml

Procedure

- Bring sections to water.
- Apply hematoxylin solution for requisite time.
- Wash briefly in water and differentiate in acid alcohol (one rapid dip).
- Wash in water and blue for 3–5 minutes.
- Observe under microscope to check the nuclei—should be deep blue with vesicular nuclei showing well-marked chromatin pattern.
- Wash well in running water and counter stain with eosin solution for 30 seconds to 1 minute.
- Wash quickly in water, dehydrate in alcohol. Clear and mount with DPX.

Observations

- Keratohyalin, nuclei, cytoplasmic RNA, some calcium salts, bacteria appear blue colour.
- Muscle, keratin, coarse elastic fibres, fibrin, fibrinoid appear deep pink/bright red in colour.
- Collagen, reticulin, myelinated nerve fibers, amyloid appear pink in colour.
- Red blood cells appear reddish orange in colour.

Giemsa Stain

- Giemsa stain is a compound stain formed by interaction of methylene blue and eosin.
- Methylene blue, on exposure to acids, alkalis and ultraviolet light, forms a number of oxidation products (methylene azures) that are responsible for giving contrasting staining reactions.
- A modified Giemsa stain, i.e. May-Grunwald Giemsa stain is used for staining of fungi.

Staining Reagents

i. *May-Grunwald stock solution*
   May-Grunwald dye   1 gm
   Methanol   300 ml

- Dissolve the May-Grunwald dye in methanol and heat up to 60°C for one hour.
- Working dilution of 1:1 is to be prepared freshly.

ii. Giemsa stock solution

Giemsa dye	1 gm
Methanol	85 ml
Glycerol	54 ml

- Mix well the ingredients.
- Working dilution of 1:9 is to be prepared freshly.

Procedure

- Prepare smear on a clean glass slide.
- Fix smears in methanol for 5 to 10 minutes.
- Apply diluted May-Grunwald stain and allow it to act for 10 minutes.
- Without washing the smear, transfer the slides to working Giemsa stain.
- Allow Giemsa stain to act for 15 minutes.
- Wash and differentiate by keeping the water on slides for 1–2 minutes until desired color balance is achieved.
- Allow it air dry, mount and observe under the microscope.

Observations

- Nuclei of the fungi appear purple in colour
- Fungal cell cytoplasm appears blue to mauve in colour
- Red blood cells appear pink in colour.

Uses

It is commonly used to demonstrate intracellular yeast cells of *Histoplasma capsulatum* and other intracellular fungi.

Periodic Acid–Schiff Stain

Principle

- Schiff reagent is a leucofuchsin—a colourless reagent formed by the reaction of basic fuchsin with sulfurous acid.
- Leucofuchsin is converted to a coloured product by aldehydes liberated from fungal cell wall by hydrolysis.

- The polysaccharides of fungi and bacteria are oxidized by periodic acid or chromic acid to yield large number of aldehyde groups because of which they stain intense red or magenta in colour with Schiff's reagent.
- The protein and nucleic acids are not stained.
- Glucan and mannan polysaccharides in the fungal cell wall are oxidized to aldehydes.

Staining Reagents

i. 1% aqueous periodic acid.
ii. Schiff's reagent

Basic fuchsin	1 gm
Potassium/sodium metabisulphite	2 gm
Concentrated hydrochloric acid	2 ml
Activated charcoal	2 gm
Distilled water	200 ml

Procedure

Preparation of smears from clinical specimens

- For preparation of smears from skin and nail scrapings, place a thin film of albumin on a clean glass slide.
- Embed several thin skin or nail scrapings in the thin film of albumin by placing them on top of the albumin and gently pressing down with another clean glass slide.
- Allow smear to air dry for several hours or alternatively slide can be placed in a slide warmer or in an incubator.
- Do not heat the smear. Fix it over a flame.
- For preparation of smears from tissue—prepare a homogenate from the tissue.
- Place a drop of homogenate in the center of a clean glass slide.
- Spread it as a thin smear.
- Allow it to air dry.
- For preparation of smears from exudates/purulent material—place a drop of water in a center glass slide.
- Emulsify a loopful of material in the water and spread across the slide.
- Allow it to air dry.

Staining Procedure

- Place smear in absolute ethanol for 1 minute.
- Drain alcohol and immediately place slide in periodic acid solution for 5 minutes to oxidize.
- Wash in running water for 2 minutes.
- Apply Schiff's reagent and allow it to act for 15 minutes.
- Wash in running tap water for 5–10 minutes. This intensifies color reaction.
- Apply hematoxylin solution to stain nuclei.
- Dehydrate in alcohol, place in xylene for 2 minutes and mount in synthetic resin medium.
- Observe under the microscope.

Observations

- Fungal elements appear—magenta/deep pink in colour
- Nuclei appear blue in colour.
- Background appears pink to red, depending on thickness of preparation.
- Bacteria and neutrophils may retain the basic fuchsin like fungal elements, but they do not interfere in interpretation of results.

Uses

This stain is useful for demonstration of fungi in tissue that are stained darker than surrounding tissues.

Disadvantages

- The important disadvantage is that many components of tissue containing carbohydrates are stained by PAS stain.
- It does not stain Actinomycetes such as *Nocardia* species.

Gridely's Fungal Stain

- This staining method is similar to PAS staining. It uses chromic acid as oxidizing agent.
- The aldehydes that are produced recolor Schiff's reagent, giving fungi purple color.
- This staining technique is a combination of Bauer, Schiff and aldehyde fuschin techniques.

Staining Reagents

- 4% aqueous chromium trioxide (chromic acid)
- Schiff's reagent
- Aldehyde fuschin solution
- Saturated tartrazine in cellosolve
- Sulphurous acid rinse
  - 10% aq. sodium metabisulphite—6 ml
  - Molar hydrochloride acid—5 ml
  - Distilled water—100 ml

Procedure

- Bring sections to water.
- Apply folic acid solution and allow it to act for 1 hour.
- Wash in tap water, then in distilled water.
- Apply Schiff's reagent for 15 minutes.
- Treat with sulphurous acid solution for three changes over 6 minutes.
- Wash in water for 10 minutes.
- Apply aldehyde fuschin solution for 20–30 minutes.
- Wash in 50% alcohol and then in water.
- Wash in absolute alcohol and stain with tartrazine solution for half to one minute.
- Wash in cellosolve, dehydrate to absolute ethyl alcohol, clear in xylene and mount in DPX mount.

Observations

- Fungi, elastin, some mucins appear purple in colour.
- Background appears yellow in colour.

Grocott-Gomori's Methenamine–Silver Nitrate Stain

Principle

- The chemical basis for the reaction depends on the availability of free aldehyde groups for the reduction of an alkaline methenamine–silver nitrate complex to metallic silver.

- The aldehydes reduce methenamine–silver nitrate. This reduction results into brown-black staining of fungal cell wall because of deposition of reduced silver.
- Reduced silver is deposited wherever the aldehydes are located in the fungal cell wall.
- These aldehydes are liberated by oxidation of the glucan and mannan polysaccharides present in the fungal cell walls.

Staining Reagents

i. *5% chromic acid solution*

Chromium trioxide	5 gm
Distilled water	100 ml

ii. *Methenamine silver nitrate solution*

5% silver nitrate	5 ml
3% methenamine	100 ml

   - Shake well to dissolve white precipitate.
   - Keep resulting clear solution at 4°C.
   - It remains stable for 1–2 months.

iii. *1% sodium bisulfite*

Sodium bisulfite	1 gm
Distilled water	100 ml

iv. *5% borax solution*

Sodium borate	5 gm
Distilled water	100 ml

Working Solution

- Borax 5% solution: 2 ml + distilled water 25 ml
- Mix and add 25 ml of stock solution
- 0.1% ferric chloride
- 1% sodium metabisulfite (aqueous)
- 5% sodium thiosulphate (aqueous)

Stock Light Green

Light green SF (yellow)	0.2 gm
Distilled water	100 ml
Glacial acetic acid	0.2 ml

- Dissolve 0.2 gm of light green in 0.2 ml glacial acetic acid and 100 ml of distilled water to make the light-green stock solution.

Working Light Green

Light green stock solution   10 ml
Distilled water   40 ml

- To make the working solution, dilute 10 ml of stock light green solution in 40 ml of distilled water.

Procedure

- Fix slide in methanol and air dry. Positive control slide must be included each time the staining procedure is performed.
- Cover slide with 5% chromic acid solution for 1 hour (to oxidize).
- Rinse in distilled water for a few seconds.
- Cover slide with 1% sodium metabisulphite for 1 min (to bleach).
- Wash in water for 5–10 minutes then in four changes of distilled water.
- Place slide in pre-heated working silver solution (pre-heated to 56°C for one hour in a Coplin jar in water bath) in a water bath at 56°C for 15 to 20 min until smeared section of the slide turns yellowish brown.

  (*Note:* The methenamine–silver nitrate solution must be freshly prepared before use and can be used only once. Other solutions may be re-used again for up to a month provided fungal contamination does not occur).
- Wash in six changes of distilled water.
- Dip slide (or flood slide on a staining rack) in a Coplin jar containing 0.1% ferric chloride for 3 minutes.
- Rinse well in water.
- Cover slide with sodium thiosulfate for 5 min (to fix).
- Rinse in distilled water for 30 seconds.
- Counter stain smear with light green working solution for 1–2 minutes.
- Wash in water.

- Dehydrate, clear and place a drop of DPX, and cover with cover slip.
- Observe under the microscope.

Observations

- Fungal hyphae and yeast bodies appear black in colour
- The cysts of *Pneumocystis jirovecii* also stain black
- Background remains green.

Mayer's Mucicarmine Stain

- This stain is used for staining of *Cryptococcus* and *Rhinosporidium* species.
- *Cryptococcus* stains deep rose red in colour, nuclei stain black in colour and tissue stains yellow in colour.
- In rhinosporidiosis, sporangium and endospores are stained by mucicarmine stain.

Staining Reagents

Carmine	1 gm
50% alcohol	100 ml
Aluminium hydroxide	1 gm
Anhydrous aluminium chloride	0.5 gm

- Grind 1 gm carmine and place in large conical flask.
- Add 100 ml of 50% alcohol and mix.
- Add 1 gm aluminium hydroxide, mix and add 0.5 gm anhydrous aluminium chloride.
- Mix and boil gently for 2.5 minutes.
- Cool and filter.
- Store at 4°C (it can be stored) for 6 months or so.

Procedure

- Bring sections to water.
- Apply alum hematoxylin solution to stain nuclei.
- Differentiate well in acid–alcohol and blue appropriately.
- Apply mucicarmine solution and allow it to act for 20 minutes.
- Wash in water, dehydrate, clear and mount.

Observations

- Mucins appear red in colour.
- Nuclei appear blue in colour.

Masson-Fontana Silver Stain (MFSS)

- Masson's technique using Fontana's silver solution is used to demonstrate substances capable of reducing silver salts to metallic silver.
- This stain is used to identify phaeoid (dematiaceous) fungi.

Staining Reagents

   i. *Silver solution*

- Add strong ammonia drop by drop to 20 ml of 10% aqueous solution of silver nitrate.
- Go on adding it until the precipitate formed just dissolves.
- A faint opalescence appears when end point is reached.
- Finally add 20 ml of distilled water, mix it well and filter.
- Store this solution in a dark container and may be used for one month.

   ii. *0.5% aqueous sodium thiosulphate*

   iii. *1% aqueous neutral red.*

Procedure

- Bring sections to distilled water.
- Apply ammoniacal silver solution in dark container (Coplin jar painted black) and allow it to act for 20–40 minutes at 56°C or overnight at room temperature.
- Wash well in several changes of distilled water.
- Treat with 0.5% sodium thiosulphate for 2 minutes. A stronger solution tends to bleach reduced silver.
- Wash and apply counter stain in neutral red solution for 3–5 minutes.
- Wash, dehydrate, clear and mount.

Observations

Melanin, argentaffin, chromaffin, some lipofuscin pigment appear black in colour and nuclei appear red in colour.

Toluidine Blue O Stain for *P. jirovecii*

Staining Reagents

i. *Sulfation reagent*

Ether	60 ml
Conc. H_2SO_4	60 ml
Distilled water	0.72 ml

- Add distilled water to ether in a flask and shake well.
- Place flask in ice water and add concentrated H_2SO_4 slowly using a separate funnel.
- Transfer reagent to jar and seal the lid.

ii. *Toluidine blue O stain*

Toluidine blue O	0.3 gm
Conc. HCl	2 ml
Absolute ethanol	140 ml
Distilled water	60 ml

- Mix toluidine blue O in distilled water.
- Add HCl and then alcohol.

Procedure

- Prepare smear on a clean glass and allow it to dry.
- Place in sulfation reagent for 5 minutes.
- Rinse slide with tap water for 1 minute.
- Stain with toluidine blue O stain for 2 minutes and wash.
- Dry slide and observe under oil immersion objective lens (100X).

Observations

- Cysts of *P. jirovecii* appear purple in colour
- Tissue remnants and debris appear blue in colour.
- Trophozoites are not discernible.

Acridine Orange Stain

The acridine orange stain has affinity for nucleic acids; hence when fungi are stained with this stain and viewed under ultraviolet light, RNA component of cells fluoresces with shades of orange and red, while DNA component gives green shades.

Staining Reagents

- 0.1% aqueous acridine orange—it is to be diluted with 10 parts of phosphate buffer to make 0.01% solution before use.
- Buffer: Phosphate buffer with pH 6.0.
- Differentiator: 0.1 M calcium chloride.

Procedure

- Bring alcohol fixed smears to distilled water.
- Rinse in 1% acetic acid for a few seconds then two changes of distilled water over one minute.
- Apply diluted acridine orange solution and allow it to act for 3 minutes.
- Rinse in phosphate buffer for 1 minute.
- Differentiate in 0.1 M calcium chloride solution for 30 seconds.
- Wash in phosphate buffer and mount in same and observe under fluorescence microscope.

Observations

- DNA appears yellow-green in colour.
- RNA and mucins appear red in colour.

Note: Formalin fixed material does not stain satisfactorily, neither does material fixed in Bouin's solution. Alcohol is fixative of choice.

Fluorescent–Antibody Staining

- This staining is important for demonstration of fungi in tissue sections or other clinical specimens.
- This method can also be used to detect fungal antigen in clinical specimens such as pus, blood, CSF, tissue impression smears and in paraffin sections of formalin fixed tissue.

Procedure

- In this staining method, the tissue section or smear of clinical specimen is fixed on a clean glass slide.
- The smear is stained with fluorescent dyes such as fluorescein isothiocyanate or lissamine rhodamine conjugated to Abs.
- Specific Ab tagged with fluorescent dye is used to locate and identify Ags in tissues.
- It is allowed to react for 30–60 minutes at 37°C and observed for fluorescence under UV microscope.

Uses

It is used for detection of fungi or their antigens in tissues, pus, blood or other specimens in various fungal infections where organisms are scanty in number.

18

Staining Procedures in Parasitology

INTRODUCTION

- As culture methods are routinely impracticable and serological methods are relatively less important in diagnosis, morphologic features for the identification of parasites forms important part in the diagnosis of parasitic infections. Hence, microscopy plays an important role in the diagnosis of parasitic diseases.
- Each parasite possesses distinctive morphological feature, hence the study of morphology is helpful in the identification of parasites.
- Different microscopic methods are routinely used for diagnosis of parasitic diseases.
- The commonly used staining methods in Parasitology are broadly classified into following two types:
  - Temporary preparations
  - Permanent stained smears

TEMPORARY PREPARATIONS

These include wet mounts:

Wet Mounts

- These are the simplest techniques most commonly used for stool examination.
- Although most commonly used for the examination of faeces, they are also used for examination of urine, blood, CSF, genital specimens, aspirates, etc. in various parasitic diseases.

- These methods are useful for demonstration of parasitic elements in stool, anal swabs, etc. in the diagnosis of intestinal parasitic diseases (stool wet mounts) (Table 18.1), for demonstration of microfilaria and tryopanosomes in blood wet mount, for demonstration of parasites causing respiratory tract infections in sputum wet mount, for demonstration of parasites causing urinary tract infections in urine wet mount, for demonstration of *Trichomonas vaginalis* in vaginal swab and urethral discharge, for

Table 18.1: Different morphological forms of parasites seen in faeces

Protozoan Parasites

Trophozoites	Cysts
Entamoeba histolytica	Entamoeba histolytica
Giardia lamblia	Giardia lamblia
Balantidium coli	Balantidium coli
	Isospora belli
	Cryptosporidium species

Helminthic Parasites

Adult worms	Eggs	Larvae
Ascaris lumbricoides	Ascaris lumbricoides	Strongyloides stercoralis
Ancylostoma duodenale	Ancylostoma duodenale	
Enterobius vermicularis	Trichuris trichiura	
Fasciolopsis buski	Necator americanus	
	Fasciolopsis buski	
Segments	Schistosoma mansoni	
Taenia saginata	Schistosoma japonicum	
Taenia solium	Fasciola hepatica	
Diphyllobothrium latum	Clonorchis sinensis	
Dipylidium caninum	Paragonimus westermani	
Hymenolepis species	Enterobius vermicularis	
	Capillaria species	
	Diphyllobothrium latum	
	Taenia saginata	
	Taenia solium	
	Hymenolepis nana	
	Hymenolepis diminuta	
	Dipylidium caninum	

demonstration of parasites in aspirated material, etc. (Table 18.2).

- These methods can be used/performed in any laboratories even at the peripheral level because of their simplicity and limited requirements.
- A wet mount can be prepared directly from specimen itself or from concentrated specimens.
- Three basic types of wet mounts used in Parasitology are:
  - Saline preparation
  - Iodine preparation and
  - Lactophenol cotton blue (LPCB) mount.

Table 18.2: Different morphological forms of parasites seen in various specimens other than faeces

- *Blood*
  - *Microfilaria* and *trypanosoma*
- *Sputum*
  - *Paragonimus westermani*—eggs
  - *Entamoeba histolytica*—trophozoites
  - *Echinococcus granulosus*—solices and hooklets
  - *Ascaris lumbricoides*—rhabditiform larvae
  - *Strongyloides stercoralis*—filariform larvae
- *Urine*
  - *Schistosoma haematobium*—eggs
  - *Wuchereria bancrofti*—microfilaria
  - *Trichomonas vaginalis*—trophozoites
- *Genital specimens*
  - *Trichomonas vaginalis*—trophozoites
- *Aspirates*
  - *Pneumocystis carinii*—lung aspirate
  - *Entamoeba histolytica*—lung and liver aspirates
  - *Echinococcus granulosus*—hydatid aspirates
  - Trypanosomes, leishmania, amoebae —lymph nodes, spleen, bone marrow, etc.
- *Cerebrospinal fluid (CSF)*
  - *Naegleria*
  - *Acanthamoeba* species
  - *Entamoeba histolytica*

SALINE PREPARATION (DIRECT WET MOUNT)

Normal Saline or Physiological Saline

Sodium chloride	9 gm
Distilled water	1000 ml

- Dissolve sodium chloride in distilled water.

Procedure

- Take a clean glass slide and put a drop of saline on it.
- With the help of applicator stick/loop/pipette, mix small amount of faecal matter (approximately 2 mg)/other specimen in a drop of normal saline to make a smooth suspension.
- Apply cover slip (22 × 22 mm) gently taking care that no air bubbles form.
- Observe under low power objective (10X) with low intensity of light then under high power objective (40X) with increased intensity of light. The intensity of light is to be adjusted according to the thickness of preparation.
- Oil immersion-routinely impracticable but can be used after sealing cover slip with paraffin, petroleum jelly or nail polish.
- *Method of examination:* The preparation should be first observed under low power objective (10X) starting from one end to another for any suspicious object and then under high power (40X) for identification/confirmation of trophozoites/ cysts/ova.

Observations

- *It is an unstained preparation:* Parasitic elements are not stained and they appear colourless.
- *As parasitic elements are live in this preparation:* Live motile trophozoites can be seen, if present.

Uses

- It is employed primarily to demonstrate
- Motile trophozoite stage of protozoan parasites
- Helminthic eggs

- Helminthic larvae
- RBCs
- WBCs
- Cysts of protozoa may also be seen.

Protozoa in Wet Mounts

- In saline mounts, trophozoites and cysts of amoebae and flagellates may be seen.
- Cysts appear as round or oval, refractile structures.
- The trophozoites of flagellates are usually pyriform (elongated, pear-shaped).
- In freshly passed faeces, motile trophozoites may be seen. Motility can be very helpful in identifying species, especially in case of flagellates.
- Organisms may be detected with the low-power (10X) objective, but a high-power objective is required for correct identification.
- High-power objective can be used to observe the motility, inclusions like erythrocytes and yeasts in amoebic trophozoites, chromatoid bodies in amoebic cysts, and the shape and structural details of flagellate trophozoites and cysts.

Worms and Larvae in Saline Mounts

- Most of the eggs are large enough to be recognized with the low-power (10X) objective, but a few small eggs require a high power objective.
- In saline mounts, larvae of *Strongyloides stercoralis* may be seen. Hookworm larvae are not usually present if the sample is fresh, but it may be necessary to distinguish between these two species if an old sample is examined.

IODINE PREPARATION

- It is a stained preparation in which iodine is used for staining parasitic elements.
- A week iodine solution, such as Lugol's iodine, Dobell and 'O' Conner's or D'Antoni's iodine is used.

Staining Reagent

Lugol' Iodine

Iodine	10 gm
Potassium iodide	20 gm
Distilled water	300 ml

- Dissolve potassium iodide in distilled water and then add iodine.
- Dissolve in distilled water.

Dobell's Iodine

Iodine	2 gm
Potassium iodide	4 gm
Distilled water	100 ml

- Dissolve potassium iodide in distilled water and then add iodine.
- Dissolve in distilled water.

D' Antoni's Iodine

Iodine	1 gm
Potassium iodide	1.5 gm
Distilled water	100 ml

- Dissolve potassium iodide in distilled water and then add iodine.
- Dissolve in distilled water.

Procedure

- It is same as saline preparation. Instead of saline, iodine solution is used.
- Take a clean glass slide and put a drop of iodine on it.
- With the help of applicator stick/loop/pipette, mix small amount of faecal matter (approximately 2 mg)/other specimen in a drop of iodine to make a smooth suspension.
- Apply cover slip (22 × 22 mm) gently taking care that no air bubbles form.
- Observe under low power objective (10X) with low intensity of light then under high power objective (40X) with increased intensity of light.

- Oil immersion-routinely impracticable but can be used after sealing cover slip with paraffin, petroleum jelly or nail polish.
- *Method of examination:* The preparation should be first observed under low power objective (10X) starting from one end to another for any suspicious object and then under high power (40X) for identification/confirmation of trophozoites/cysts/ova.

Observations (Fig. 18.1)

- Cytoplasm of the cysts appears yellow or light brown
- Nuclei appear dark brown
- The peripheral chromatoid bodies appear light yellow and may not be very clear
- Glycogen mass in young cysts appears dark brown with iodine.

Uses

- This preparation is used mainly to stain glycogen and the nuclei of cysts specifically used for demonstration of cystic stage.
- Trophozoite stage can also be demonstrated.
- Eggs and larvae can also be demonstrated but as iodine stains non-bile stained eggs also, hence less important as far as

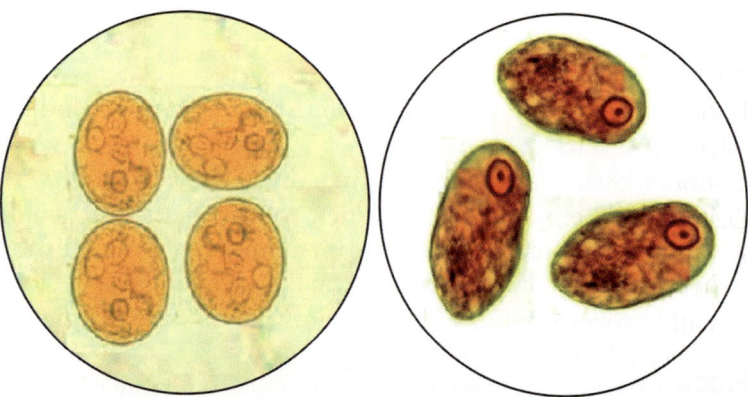

Fig. 18.1: Iodine preparation showing *Entamoeba coli*—cysts and trophozoites

differentiation of bile stained and non-bile stained eggs are concerned.

LACTOPHENOL COTTON BLUE (LPCB) MOUNT

- LPCB mount using LPCB is a commonly used method in a mycology laboratory for the demonstration of fungi and fungal elements.
- It is also used for the wet mount of stool preparation to demonstrate intestinal parasites.
- LPCB is a combined fixative, staining, and clearing agent. It contains the cotton blue that stains the intestinal protozoa and helminthic eggs deep blue in colour. It contains phenol and lactic acid that kill viable fungi. Glycerol in the LPCB stain provides a semi-permanent preparation.
- In this wet-mount preparation, the protozoal cysts and helminthic eggs are stained deep blue in colour. The LPCB stains the internal structures of trophozoites, cysts, and ova; thus, facilitating their recognition and identification in stool specimens.
- The most important advantage of LPCB is that it can be used for the demonstration of the intestinal coccidian parasites such as Cyclospora and Isospora in stool specimens.

Staining Reagents

LPCB

Melted phenol crystals	20 ml
Lactic acid	20 ml
Glycerol	40 ml
Cotton blue	0.050 or 0.075 gm
Distilled water	20 ml

- Mix well all the reagents properly and dissolve 0.050 gm or 0.075 gm of cotton blue stain in distilled water before mixing with remaining reagents.

Procedure

- It is same as saline or iodine preparation. Instead of saline or iodine, LPCB solution is used.

- Take a clean glass slide and put a drop of LPCB on it.
- With the help of applicator stick, mix small amount of faecal matter in a drop of LPCB to make a smooth suspension.
- Apply cover slip (22 × 22 mm) gently taking care that no air bubbles form.
- Observe under low power objective (10X) with low intensity of light then under high power objective (40X) with increased intensity of light.
- *Method of examination:* The preparation should be first observed under low power objective (10X) starting from one end to another for any suspicious object and then under high power (40X) for identification/confirmation. Observe at least for 30 minutes.

Observations

- Cytoplasm-appears deep blue in colour.
- Nucleus/nuclei-appear blue in colour.

EOSIN MOUNT

The eosin mount is used for the detection of motile trophozoites of *Entamoeba* species.

Staining Reagents

Eosin in saline solution

Procedure

- It is same as saline or iodine preparation. Instead of saline or iodine, eosin solution is used.
- Take a clean glass slide and put a drop of warm (37°C) solution of eosin in saline on it.
- With the help of applicator stick, mix small amount of faecal matter in a drop of eosin and emulsify to make a smooth suspension.
- Apply cover slip (22 × 22 mm) gently taking care that no air bubbles form.
- Observe under low power objective (10X) with low intensity of light then under high power objective (40X) with increased intensity of light.

- *Method of examination:* The preparation should be first observed under low power objective (10X) starting from one end to another for any suspicious object and then under high power (40X) for identification/confirmation.

Observations

- The amoebae are easily seen unstained against a pink background.
- The coarse, granular endoplasm can be differentiated from the clear, colourless ectoplasm.

BUFFERED METHYLENE BLUE (BMB) MOUNT

The BMB mount is used for the detection of trophozoites of *Entamoeba* species.

Staining Reagents

BMB

Procedure

- It is same as saline or iodine preparation. Instead of saline or iodine, BMB solution is used.
- Observe under low power objective (10X) with low intensity of light then under high power objective (40X) with increased intensity of light.

Observations

- The trophozoites of amoebae may remain motile for 5–10 minutes.
- Trophozoites are stained light blue in colour.
- Inclusions in the cytoplasm are stained deep blue in colour.
- Cysts are not stained.

PERMANENT PREPARATIONS

- Permanent staining techniques are not used routinely and are not required for the identification of worm eggs or larvae.

- Permanently stained preparations are occasionally required for the following purposes:
  - For identification of oocysts of cryptosporidium;
  - For identification of protozoan trophozoites, in case of doubt;
  - For confirmation of the identity of protozoan cysts, where doubt exists;
  - For keeping a permanent record;
  - For sending to a reference laboratory for an expert opinion.
- These staining techniques include:

Modified Ziehl-Neelsen Techniques

Staining Reagents
- Carbol fuchsin
- 5% aqueous sulphuric acid
- 0.3% methylene blue.

Hot Modified Acid-fast Staining Method

Procedure
- A faecal smear is prepared on a glass slide.
- The smear is fixed by heat at 70°C for 10 minutes.
- The heat-fixed slide is kept on the staining rack and smear is covered with carbol fuchsin.
- The slide is heated from below till carbol fuschin starts steaming.
- The slide is allowed to stain for 9 minutes. If needed, more carbol fuchsin is added to prevent slides from drying.
- The slide is rinsed with water.
- The smear is decolourised with 5% aqueous sulphuric acid for 30 seconds.
- The smear is then washed with tap water or distilled water.
- The counter stain-methylene blue is applied and allowed to act for 1 minute.
- The smear is washed with tap water or distilled water, then the water is drained off and dried.
- Observe under oil immersion lens (100X).

Observations

- The acid-fast *Cryptosporidium* appears pink in colour
- Non-acid-fast structures and background appear blue.

Kinyoun's Cold Stain Method (for *Cryptosporidium* spp.)

- Cover smear with Kinyoun's carbol fuchsin stain. Keep it for 5 minutes without heating. Rinse slide with distilled water.
- Decolorize with acid-alcohol (3 ml of HCl + 97 ml of 95% alcohol) for 3 minutes. Rinse with distilled water.
- Repeat decolourization until no red color appears in the wash. Rinse with distilled water.
- Counter stain with methylene blue for 1 minute. Rinse slide with distilled water. Air dry. Do not blot.
- Observe under oil immersion lens (100X).

Observations

- The acid-fast *Cryptosporidium* appears pink in colour
- Non-acid-fast structures and background appear blue.

Safranin-methylene Blue Technique

Staining Reagents

- Hydrochloric acid-methanol solution
- Safranin solution
- 1% (w/v) Methylene blue-phosphate solution.

Procedure

- Prepare a thin smear of faeces.
- Allow it to air-dry and then pass the slide once through the flame of a spirit lamp.
- Fix the smear in hydrochloric acid-methanol solution for 4 minutes.
- Wash with clean tap-water.
- Apply 1% aqueous safranin solution to smear. Heat the stain by holding a lightened spirit swab under the slide. Do not let the stain dry on the smear. Allow it to act for 1 minute.

- Wash off the stain with clean tap-water.
- Counter stain smear with methylene blue solution and allow it to act for 30 seconds.
- Wash with clean tap-water and dry the slide.
- Scan smear for oocysts under high power objective (40X) and use oil immersion (100X) objective to identify oocysts.

Observations

- Cryptosporidium oocysts are round to oval orange-pink bodies (4–6 μm diameter).
- The sporozoites within the oocysts stain slightly darker.

Trichrome Stain

Staining Reagent

Trichrome stain

Chromotrope	0.6 gm
Light green SF	0.3 gm
Phosphotungstic acid	0.7 gm
Glacial acetic acid	1 ml
Distilled water	100 ml

- Mix all constituents with glacial acetic acid.
- Allow this mixture to stand for 15 to 30 minutes.
- Add distilled water to this mixture.
- Store this reagent in coloured bottle.

D' Antoni's Iodine

Procedure

- Prepare smear from the fresh or PVA-preserved stool sample on a clean glass slide.
- In case of fresh faecal smear, the slide is placed in 70% ethanol for 1 minute for fixing.
- The slide is placed in 70% ethanol and D' Antoni's iodine for 2–5 minutes.
- Ethanol is changed two times, one for 5 minutes and the other for 2–5 minutes.
- The slide is removed and then placed in trichrome stain solution for 10 minutes.

- The slide is dipped in just for 3 seconds in the mixture of 90% ethanol and 1% acetic acid.
- Then, the slide is dipped once in 100% ethanol. The 100% ethanol is changed two times, one for 2 minutes and the other for 3 minutes.
- The slide is then placed in xylene first for 2 minutes and then xylene is changed, after which it is placed for 5 minutes.
- The stained smear is mounted in a mounting medium (e.g. permount) using a No. 1 thickness cover glass.
- Observe under the oil immersion lens (100X).

Observations

- Trophozoites as well as cysts of protozoan parasites are stained.
- Cytoplasm appears greenish-blue or green in colour.
- Nuclei, chromatoid bodies and filaments of flagella appear red or purple in colour.
- Inclusions such as red blood cells, bacteria, etc. appear red or purple in colour.

Modified Trichrome Stain

- It is modified by Weber et al. in 1992.
- It is used for staining of faecal smears or duodenal aspirates.

Staining Reagent

Modified trichrome stain

Chromotrope 2R	6 gm
Fast green FCF	0.15 gm
12-tungstophosphoric acid	0.7 gm
Glacial acetic acid	3 ml
Distilled water	100 ml

- Mix all constituents with glacial acetic acid.
- Allow this mixture to stand for 30 minutes.
- Add distilled water to this mixture.
  - Acid-alcohol mixture

90% Ethanol	995.5 ml
Glacial acetic acid	4.5 ml

Procedure

- Make a suspension of liquid stool or duodenal aspirate in 10% formalin in a 1:3 ratio.
- Spread about 10 µl aliquot over an area of about 1 cm² on a clean glass slide.
- Allow it to dry.
- Fix in methanol for 5 minutes.
- Apply modified trichrome stain and allow it to act for 90 minutes.
- Rinse briefly in ethanol (95%) for 3 seconds.
- Ethanol (95%) for 5 minutes.
- Ethanol (100%) for 5 minutes.
- Xylene 3 minutes (two changes).
- Mount in DPX and observe under oil immersion lens (100X).

Iron Haematoxylin Stain

Staining Reagents

i. Schaudinn's fluid

Saturated mercuric chloride (aqueous solution)	40 ml
Absolute ethanol	20 ml
Glacial acetic acid	3 ml

ii. Mordant solution (4% aqueous solution of ferric ammonium sulphate)

Ferric ammonium sulphate	4 gm
Distilled water	100 ml

- Use freshly prepared solution

iii. Haematoxylin

Haematoxylin	5 gm
Absolute ethanol	10 ml
Distilled water	100 ml

- Store in a clear glass stoppered bottle for ripening by exposure to sunlight before use.

Staining Procedure

- Prepare smear on a clean glass slide by spreading stool sample with wooden applicator stick as evenly as possible.
- Fix smear immediately in Schaudinn's fluid for 30 minutes.
- Treat smear with 50% ethanol for 5 minutes.
- Treat smear with 70% ethanol for 5 minutes.
- Apply iodine solution in 70% ethanol for 5 minutes.
- Apply 70% ethanol two changes 10 minutes each.
- Apply 50% ethanol for 5 minutes.
- Apply 30% ethanol for 5 minutes.
- Distilled water-two changes—5 minutes each.
- Place slide in mordant solution for 4 hours.
- Rinse in distilled water.
- Stain with haematoxylin for 4 hours.
- Treat with distilled water for 2 minutes.
- Differentiate in 1% ferric ammonium sulphate, repeatedly checking differentiation by microscopy and stopping differentiation, when sufficient, by washing in distilled water.
- Dehydrate in ascending concentrations of ethanol, clear in xylene and mount in DPX.
- Observe under oil immersion lens (100X).

METHODS FOR STAINING BLOOD FILMS

- Examination of blood is an important part in the diagnosis of those parasitic infections, in which the parasite itself or in any stage of its development, circulates in the bloodstream.
- Parasites found in blood include:
  - *Plasmodium spp.* inside the red blood cells
  - *Trypanosoma spp.* in the blood plasma
  - *W. bancrofti* in the blood plasma
  - *Brugia malayi* in the blood plasma
  - *Loa loa*–in the blood plasma
  - *Mansonella* spp. in the blood plasma
- Microscopic examination of permanent stained blood smears is essential for the accurate identification of blood parasites.

- The commonly used staining methods for examination of blood in Parasitology are of two types:
  a. Temporary preparations
  b. Permanent stained smears.

Temporary Preparations

Wet Mount

Procedure

- A drop of blood collected by finger prick is taken on a clean glass slide.
- A cover slip is applied.
- The preparation is observed first under 10X and then under 40X.

Uses

Direct wet mount of blood is used for detection of microfilaria and trypanosoma for their characteristic shape and motility.

Permanent Stained Smears

- Permanent stained smears are necessary for the specific identification of the causative agent.
- Two types of blood smears—thick and thin smears are used for the diagnosis.
  a. *Thick smear* allows examination of larger amount of blood, which increases the possibility of detecting light infections.
  b. *Thin smears* helps in species identification.
- Thick and thin smears are made from peripheral blood and stained with Romanowsky's stains.

ROMANOWSKY'S STAINS

- These are differential stains with combination of methylene blue and eosin.
- They also contain oxidation products of methylene blue called azures.
- These azures provide further contrast in smears of peripheral blood stained by Romanowsky's stains.

- These stains include:
  - Leishman's stain commonly used
  - Giemsa stain
  - Wright's stain
  - Field's stain
  - JSB stain (Singh and Bhattacharji)
- Stock solutions of these stains are prepared by dissolving the stains in pure methanol.
- There are two types of theses stains
  1. Stock solution diluted with water—stock solution of some stains like Giemsa, JSB and Field's stain are diluted with distilled water (pH 7 to 7.2) before use.
  2. Stock solution not diluted with water—stock solution of some stains like Leishman's is not diluted with distilled water before use.
- The pre-treatment of peripheral blood smear differs according to the type of Romanowsky stain used (Table 18.3).
- The details of Romanowsky stains are given in Chapter 8.

HAEMATOXYLIN STAIN

It is used for demonstration of microfilariae.

Procedure

- Prepare a thick and thin blood smears on a clean glass slide by taking known amount of blood.
- Allow it to dry in air, preferably overnight.
- Flood smear with distilled water to dehaemoglobinize the smear.
- When smear becomes completely colourless, dry it in air.
- Fix with methyl alcohol for 1 minute and dry in air.
- Apply hot Harris haematoxylin (not boiling) stain and allow it to act for 7–10 minutes.
- Wash off the stain in running tap water and observe slide (still it is wet) under the microscope to check the staining of nuclei. If nuclei are understained, add hot haematoxylin stain and allow it to act for a few minutes. If overstained, i.e. the

Table 18.3: Pre-treatment of peripheral smear differs according to the type of Romanowsky stain

Stain	Specimen	Pre-treatment
1. Water based stain- distilled water is used for dilution (e.g. Giemsa, JSB, Field's)	Thin blood film and tissue smear	Methanol fixation
	Thick blood films	None
2. Methanol based stain- distilled water is not used for dilution (e.g. Leishman's)	Thin blood film and tissue smear	None
	Thick blood film	Dehaemoglobinise

nuclei are appearing as undifferentiated mass, differentiate with acid alcohol (1% HCl in 70% alcohol) for 10 seconds. Wash in water and observe. Repeat the process if necessary.

- Wash slide with running tap water (slightly alkaline in nature) for a few minutes to blue the nuclei.
- Allow smear to dry and then observe under 10X and 40X.
- As the known quantity of blood is observed, the number of microfilariae per ml of blood can be counted.

19

Staining Methods in Virology

- As cultivation of viruses is difficult and time-consuming, the isolation and identification of viruses is not routinely practicable.
- Hence, serological tests and direct demonstration of virus particles and their components are used for diagnosing viral diseases.
- Serological tests are more commonly used for diagnosis than microscopic methods.
- Different microscopic methods used in the diagnosis of viral diseases are as follows:
  1. Demonstration of cytopathic changes in infected host cells, e.g. Tzanck cells in herpes simplex virus.
  2. Demonstration of virus inclusion bodies by Giemsa or eosin methylene blue stain.
  3. Demonstration of virus by direct immunofluorescence stain.
  4. Demonstration of virus by electron microscope or immunoelectron microscopy.

1. DEMONSTRATION OF CYTOPATHIC CHANGES IN INFECTED HOST CELLS

- This is the most commonly used method for demonstration of Tzanck cells.
- Tzanck smear is used for demonstration of Tzanck cells.
- It is a very simple and rapid technique.

Preparation of Smear

- In viral infections, to obtain accurate results, smear is prepared from the scrapings obtained from the base of fresh vesicles, rather than crusted one.
- The base of a fresh vesicle is scraped with the help of a scalpel or a spatula.
- The material is then transferred to a clean glass slide and smear is prepared.
- Allow it to dry in air and stain.
- Stain it with Giemsa stain.
- Alternatively, smear can be stained with wright stain, 1 % toluidine blue, methylene blue, haematoxylin and eosin stain, and papanicolaou stain.
- When it is to be stained by Papanicolaou stain, the smear should be immediately fixed in alcohol.

Giemsa's Stain

Procedure

- The Giemsa stain solution is diluted 1:10 with distilled water.
- The smear is covered with diluted solution of Giemsa stain and it is allowed to act for 15 minutes.
- The smear is washed with water.
- The smear is allowed to dry and then observed under the microscope.

Observations

- Nuclei appear reddish blue to purple in colour.
- The cytoplasm appears blue in colour.

Uses

- It is most commonly used for demonstration of Tzanck cells (the multinucleated syncytial giant cells with faceted nuclei and homogenously stained ground glass chromatin) in infections caused by herpes simplex virus.
- It is also used in the diagnosis of herpes-zoster virus infections in which multinucleated giant cells are demonstrated by using haematoxylin and eosin staining.

- Tzanck smear can also be used for demonstration of intracytoplasmic molluscum bodies in molluscum contagiosum.
- The method can also be used in the diagnosis of vaccinia, Orf, milker's nodules and variola viruses.

Papanicolaou Stain

- Papanicolaou stain (also known as PAP stain) is the most important and most commonly used staining method in cytopathology.
- It is a polychromatic stain containing multiple staining agents to differentially stain various components of the cells.
- This technique was developed by George Papanicolaou, the father of cytopathology.
- Papanicolaou stain includes both acidic and basic dyes.
- Acidic dye stains the basic components of the cell and basic dye stain the acidic components of the cell.
- The polychromatic PAP stain uses **five dyes in three solutions**.

  1. **Hematoxylin:** It is the nuclear stain which stains cell nuclei blue. It has affinity for chromatin, attached to sulphate groups on the DNA.
  2. **Orange Green 6:** This is the first acidic counter stain (cytoplasmic stain) which stains matured and keratinized cells. The target structures are stained orange in different intensities.
  3. **Eosin Azure:** This is the second counter stain which is a polychrome mixture of eosin Y, light green SF and Bismarck brown.
     - **Eosin Y** gives a pink colour to cytoplasm of mature squamous cells, nucleoli, cilia and red blood cells.
     - **Light green SF** stains blue to cytoplasm of metabolically active cells like parabasal squamous cells, intermediate squamous cells and columnar cells.
     - **Bismarck brown Y** stains nothing and sometimes it is often omitted.

Staining Reagents

i. *Harris's hematoxylin (modified)*

Hematoxylin crystals	5.0 gm
Absolute alcohol	50 ml
Ammonium or potassium alum	100 ml
Distilled water	1000 ml
Mercuric chloride	2.5 gm

ii. *Orange G6 (OG 6)*

Orange G6	05 gm
95% ethyl alcohol	100 ml
Phosphotungstic acid	0.015 gm

iii. *Eosin–Azure 50 (EA 50) or Eosin–Azure 36 (EA 36)*

a. Light green SF

Light green SF yellowish	0.5 gm
95% ethyl alcohol	100 ml

b. Eosin yellow

Eosin yellow	0.5 gm
95% ethyl alcohol	100 ml

- The working solution of EA 36 is prepared as follows:

Light green SF yellowish (A)	45 ml
Eosin yellow (B)	45 ml
Phosphotungstic acid	0.200 gm

- Mix and store in refrigerator.

Procedure

- Prepare smear on a clean glass slide immediately after collection of specimen.
- Fix smear immediately while still it is wet using equal parts of ether and 95% alcohol. It may take 30 minutes to one week for fixation of smear.
- After fixation, transfer smear immediately without drying from ether–alcohol solution to 95% alcohol, then through the 80% alcohol, 70% alcohol, and water and finally to distilled water.
- Apply Harris's hematoxylin to smear and allow it to act for 8 minutes.

- Rinse gently in tap water to prevent cells from being washing off.
- Dip slide in 1% hydrochloric acid in 70% alcohol.
- Place slide under running tap water for 5 minutes to wash out the acid thoroughly.
- Observe smear under the microscope to check the proper staining of nuclei-if over stained decolourize smear with acid-alcohol and if pale in colour, reapply the hematoxylin.
- Dehydrate through distilled water and alcohol solutions. Transfer slide through 70%, 80% and 95% alcohol solutions.
- Apply OG 6 for 2 minutes.
- Rinse smear for 5 times–twice in 95% alcohol, once in 1% acetic acid in 95% alcohol, once in 1% phosphotungstic acid in 95% alcohol and once in 95% alcohol.
- Apply EA 36 or EA 50 for 3 minutes.
- Rinse smear for 9 times–3 changes of 95% alcohol, two changes of absolute alcohol and 4 changes of xylene.
- Mount in DPX and observe under the microscope.

Observations
- Nuclei appear blue in colour.
- Cytoplasm shows varying shades of pink, blue, yellow, green-grey.

Uses
- It is used for demonstration of cytopathic changes in infected host cells in different viral infections.
- It is mainly used to differentiate cells in the smear preparation of various gynecological specimens (pap smears), materials containing exfoliative cells and material from fine needle aspiration.

2. DEMONSTRATION OF VIRUS INCLUSION BODIES
- Inclusion bodies are virus—specific intracellular globular masses that are produced during the replication of virus in host cells.

- The inclusions may be crystalline aggregates of virions or made-up of virus antigens present at the site of virus synthesis.
- These are the structures with distinct size, shape location and staining properties.
- These structures can be demonstrated in virus-infected host cells under the light microscope.
- These inclusions are seen in cytoplasm, nucleus or both in the cytoplasm and the nucleus.
- The details are as follows:
  - Cytoplasmic,
  - Intranuclear, or
  - Both cytoplasmic and intranuclear

Cytoplasmic (Intracytoplasmic) Inclusions

- These are produced by viruses that assemble in the cytoplasm.
- These are mainly produced by RNA viruses and include following:
  i. **Negri bodies** are the eosinophilic inclusion bodies in the cytoplasm of the brain cells infected by rabies virus. Their demonstration helps in the presumptive diagnosis of rabies.
  ii. **Guarnieri bodies** are small multiple inclusions seen in cells infected with vaccinia virus.
  iii. **Molluscum bodies** are very large 20–30 μ in size; hence, readily seen under the low power microscope. These are seen in cells infected by *M. contagiosum*.
  iv. **Bollinger bodies:** These are inclusions seen in cells infected with fowlpox virus.

Intranuclear Inclusion Bodies

- These are the inclusion bodies produced by viruses that assemble in the nucleus of the host cells.
- These are usually produced by DNA viruses.

- These are of two types:
  1. **Cowdry type A**—These are the inclusions of variable size and have a granular appearance. These are produced by herpesvirus and yellow fever virus.
  2. **Cowdry type B**—These are circumscribed and often multiple. These are produced by adenovirus and poliovirus.

Both Cytoplasmic and Intranuclear Inclusion Bodies

- These are the inclusion bodies produced by measles virus.
- Measles virus is an RNA virus.
- The inclusion granules are generally acidophilic-stain pink when stained with Giemsa or eosin methylene blue stains.
- Some viruses form basophilic inclusions, e.g. adenovirus inclusion bodies. These are stained by haematoxylin.
- Their demonstration helps in the diagnosis of some viral infections, e.g. demonstration of Negri bodies in the cytoplasm of brain cells helps in the presumptive diagnosis of rabies.

Demonstration of Negri Bodies

- Negri bodies produced by rabies viruses in the cytoplasm of infected nerve cells or cell cultures can be detected histopathologically by microscopy or by the fluorescent antibody (FA) test.
- Seller's stain is used for staining of Negri bodies.

Staining Reagents

   i. *Methylene blue*

Methylene blue	10 g
Methanol (absolute acetone-free)	1000 ml

  ii. *Basic fuchsin*

Basic fuchsin	5 g
Methanol (absolute acetone-free)	500 ml

      Working solution

Methylene blue	2 parts
Basic fuschin	1 part

Preparation of Smears

The following methods are used for smear preparation:

i. *Impression method*

- A clean glass slide is touched against the cut surface of the section and pressed gently downwards with just enough pressure exerted to create a slight spread of the exposed surface of the tissue against the slide.
- Around 3–4 impressions can be made on one slide.
- While still moist, the slide is flooded with Seller's stain for a few seconds, rinsed under the tap and dried at room temperature without blotting.
- It is observed directly under the oil immersion lense or covered with a cover-slip mounted in Canada balsam.

ii. *Smear method*

- Place a very small section of brain on one end of the slide.
- Crush the section of tissue with the help of another slide against the first slide and then draw across the length of the slide.
- This results in a fairly homogeneous thin film of tissue covering about three-quarters of the area of the slide.

iii. *Rolling method*

Rolling technique, consists of cutting a piece of brain tissue about 5 mm in diameter, and rolling or teasing it gently over the entire surface of the slide with a toothpick or wooden applicator.

Staining Procedure

- Prepare smears or impressions using clean glass slides.
- Do not fix smears.
- Immediately, while the preparation is still moist, immerse it in the staining solution for 1–5 seconds, depending on the thickness of the smear.
- Rinse quickly in running tap water, and air-dry without blotting.
- Observe under the oil immersion lens.

Observations

- The Negri bodies appear magenta (heliotrope) to bright red in colour with well-defined dark-blue to black basophilic inner bodies.
- All parts of the nerve cell appear blue in colour and the interstitial tissue appear pink in colour.
- Erythrocytes appear copper red in colour.

3. DEMONSTRATION OF VIRUS BY DIRECT IMMUNOFLUORESCENCE STAIN

Direct immunofluorescense stain is used for demonstration of virus particles by detecting cell associated antigens.

- In this method, fluorescein isothiocyanate is conjugated with antibody that recognizes the viral antigen in specimen.
- The details are described in **chapter 16.**
- In virology, this method is used for detection viruses causing cutaneous, respiratory, ocular, and infections of bloodstream.

4. DEMONSTRATION OF VIRUS BY ELECTRON MICROSCOPY OR IMMUNOELECTRON MICROSCOPY

A. Demonstration of Virus by Electron Microscopy

- Occasionally electron microscopy can be used for direct demonstration of virus particles in specimens, especially for detection of non-cultivable and slow growing viruses present in clinical specimens.
- Viruses can be demonstrated by electron microscopy by two different techniques:
  a. Negative staining
  b. Positive staining

Negative Staining Technique

Procedure

- Place a drop of specimen (cell culture fluid or faecal extracts) on a flat piece of Parafilm.
- Invert a coated grid (400 mesh nickel grids with a pariodion film reinforced with a carbon layer) over the specimen for 2–3 minutes.

- Remove the grid from specimen and remove excess liquid by touching the edge of the grid to the top edge of a sheet of filter paper.
- Wash the grid in a slow stream of distilled water.
- Remove excess liquid as above.
- Apply a drop of staining solution–2% phosphotungstate (PTA) or 2% uranyl acetate to the grid for 1–2 minutes.
- After drying, the specimen is ready to be introduced into the electron beam.
- Sometimes, highly purified virus preparations are unable to adhere to the quoted grid. In such instances, highly purified virus preparations are mixed with bovine serum albumin (100 µg/ml) or bacitracin (20 µg/ml) before loading the preparation on the grid.
- Alternatively, before staining, the coated grids can be charged with antibody, if a specific antigen target is known.

Positive Staining Technique

- The positive staining technique is used for enhancing the contrast of virus particles.
- Using this technique, the samples are incubated in heavy metal salt solutions that react with virus particles.
- Uranyl acetate and lead citrate are the most commonly used salts.
- Grids containing ultra-thin sections of a sample are incubated for 15 minutes in uranyl acetate in dark.
- The grids are washed in distilled water and incubated in lead citrate for 4–5 minutes in absence of CO_2. NaOH tablets are used to keep the environment free from reacting with CO_2.
- At the end of the procedure the grids are washed in distilled water, air dried and observed under electron microscope.

B. Immunoelectron Microscopy

- Ab combining with viral particles causes clumping of viruses, which can be visualized by electron microscope.
- This method is used for viruses such as Hepatitis-A virus and viruses causing diarrhoea.

- The virus particles are bound to the grid and then stained with primary antibodies, which are then detected using gold-conjugated antibodies.

Procedure

- Absorb the specimen on the coated grids as described above.
- Block with 1% sterile bovine serum albumin in PBS for 2 minutes.
- Float the grid on a drop of primary antibody diluted in bovine serum albumin/PBS and incubate at room temperature for 1 hour.
- Rinse the grid in bovine serum albumin/PBS, then incubate for 1 hour in gold-conjugated secondary antibody.
- Rinse as above in PBS only, then fix in 2.5% glutaraldehyde, rinse in distilled water (3 × 1 minute) and then stain with uranyl acetate or potassium phosphotungstate.

Particle Quantification

- It may be possible to quantify virus particles by using electron microscope.
- One can determine the concentration/number of virus particles in specimens and also to estimate the particle: infectivity ratio.
- For this, a fix quantity of the specimen containing virus particles is mixed with an equal volume of latex spheres of known concentration.
- This mixture is adsorbed onto a quoted grid and stained.
- The ratio of virus particles—latex spheres is determined.
- Based on this the virus particles in given specimen are quantified.

Bibliography

1. Basic Medical Laboratory Methods in Parasitology. WHO, 1991.
2. Collee JG, Fraser AG, Marmion BP, Simmons A. Mackie and McCartney Practical Medical Microbiology. 14th ed. New Delhi: Churchill Livingstone–Elsevier, 2011.
3. Forbes BA, Sahm DF, Weissfeld AS. Bailey and Scott's Diagnostic Microbiology. 12th ed. Missouri:Mosby-Elsevier, 2007.
4. Gilkes MJ, Smith CH, Sowa J. Staining of the inclusion bodies of trachoma and inclusion conjunctivitis. Br J Ophth 1958;42:473–477.
5. Jagdish Chander. Textbook of Medical Mycology. 3rd ed. New Delhi; Mehata Publishers, 2011:514–521
6. Luna, lee G. Histopathologic methods and colour atlas of special stains and Tissue artifacts; American histolabs, Inc. publications division, Gaithersburg, MD. P. 236.
7. Monica Cheesbrough. District Laboratory Practice in Tropical Countries. 2nd ed. Part I. New Delhi: Cambridge University Press, 2009.
8. Monica Cheesbrough. District Laboratory Practice in Tropical Countries. 2nd ed. Part II. New Delhi: Cambridge University Press, 2006.
9. Nagoba BS, et al. Vital staining method–a modification of hanging drop preparation for study of bacterial motility. Ind J Med Microbiol 1991;09:32–33.
10. Nagoba BS, Pichare AP. Medical Microbiology and Parasitology: Prep Manual for Under Graduates. 3rd ed. New Delhi; Elsevier, 2016.
11. Nagoba BS, Pichare AP. Medical Parasitology: Prep Manual for Under Graduates. 2nd ed. New Delhi; Elsevier, 2012.
12. Parija SC. Textbook of Practical Microbiology. New Delhi; Ahuja Publishing House, 2012.

13. Parija SC. Textbook of Practical Paraitology. 2nd ed. New Delhi; All India Publishers, 2004.

14. Sonnenwirth AC, Jarett L. Gradwohl's Clinical Laboratory Methods and Diagnosis. 8th ed. Vol II. London:Mosby, 1980.

15. Vasantakumari R. Practical Microbiology. New Delhi: B I Publications, 2009.

16. Vedpathak DV, et al. Negative staining for bacterial motility. Ind J Med Microbiol 1995; 13: 27–28.

Index

Reader's Notes

Reader's Notes

Reader's Notes

_____

_____

_____

_____

_____

_____

_____

_____

_____

_____

_____

_____

_____

_____

_____

_____

_____

_____

_____

_____

_____

_____

_____

_____

_____

_____

_____

_____